CAN'T HOLD ME DOWN!

JOE PETRONE

ISBN: 978-0-557-09051-8

CONTENTS:

Heroes are the meek and weak,
At birth, parents will shriek.
Medical prognosis Oh so bleak,
First impression, nature's freak.

Future progress, Oh so steep,
Daily care and love, no sleep.
Parents' rejoice, with every leap,
Love for the child, Oh, so deep.

Devastation, depression, on a high,
All future visions, with a why?

Progress and outcome, bright today,
For a child, so many cast away.
He is a man now, proud and bold,
He shows the world, hate is old.

He strives and thrives, his story told,
Family, friends, love, are pure as gold.

INTRODUCTION

This book is not about the biology of Down Syndrome and the genetic disruptions caused by defective chromosomal sequences, rather it is about the reality of a child born with Downs' and his many positive God-given gifts. This story reveals the abundance of love, care and devotion needed to raise a child born with Downs'. They need the opportunity to develop as normally as possible, to acquire the emotional, mental and physical tools that are required in the world of "normal" as we know it and perceive it. This is a summary of how a loving human being is placed on this earth with a lifetime fight to change stereotypes and ancient misconceptions. This is a story of what the potential future is for a child with Down syndrome. This book will attempt to illustrate not what a Downs' child is at birth, but what he can be with the dedication and unconditional love of parents, siblings, relatives, friends and a compassionate society.

It's also about the unconditional love and affection that illuminated and radiates from within the very soul of these children, and, if given the opportunity, a flicker of hope, a
shade of respect that should be afforded to all individuals regardless of colour, creed, religion, physical appearance and

mental ability, these children can thrive amongst our so called "normal" society.

JOSH'S HUMOR

Josh is assisting at the hockey program for St. Albert Junior High. He worked daily with his coach Mr. Gaicobbo retrieving pucks, sticks, passing out the water and any other chore required. He enjoyed and still enjoys the work. One day during one of his floor hockey games Josh was hit by a stick to his groin area. He quickly folded over the pain and some attention had to be given, especially since Josh is a master of theatrics. As I approached his vicinity, which in most cases he resented during games, I asked him what was wrong. He quickly replied "he hit me in my family jewels". We all started to laugh at his response and I asked him, "Where did you learn to say that specifically?" He replied, "All the hockey players say that when they get hit in the groin by the puck, during our hockey academy". On another front, prior to going to the arena every day, I dropped Josh off at the school where Jeff Giacobbo then took him to the hockey rink for their official practices. One day he waited for Jeff in his office, Josh decided to use Jeff's cell phone. He called one of his favorite brothers-in-law at work, *which he often did. During the conversation, Chris, our son-in-law, asked him where he was calling from. Josh replied that he was calling from Jeff's office. Chris asked him if he was using Jeff's cell phone and Josh acknowledged that fact. Chris explained to Josh that he should use the land line as it is rather expensive to use the cell. Josh agreed and was ready to place the cell phone back where he found it. When Jeff walked in and saw what had happened, Jeff explained to Josh that he owed him $.75 cents for the call, and kiddingly told Josh that he wanted the money back. Without hesitation, Josh answered, "take it out of my ass" Jeff, was taken back and uncertain how to answer, decided at least to speak with Josh, as to what he had said, knowing full well that Josh did not understand his wit, sarcasm, or the inappropriateness of what he had said. Josh apologized to Jeff and nothing else was said. As Jeff walked away, he started to laugh and could not wait to call Chris, his best friend, and tell him what Josh had said. They both had a laugh and from that day Jeff recounts that story to all who ask about Josh.*

CHAPTER
1

March 15, 1985
The Beginning

When I was young, I had the opportunity to play professional soccer and football at the highest level. I played soccer with Canada's National team, and the Ital-Canadians of the Alberta Major Soccer League. In football I played at the Idaho State University, University of Calgary, University of Alberta, and with the Dallas Cowboys of the NFL (with whom I spent a brief amount of time). During this time, I visited schools and hospitals to sign autographs for many children. I spoke with several mentally and physically handicapped children. I never imagined that someday *I would be at the hospital signing documents for a mentally handicapped child of my own.* How could this be, I thought. I was not sick. I had no deformities and was normal in every way. "How could God do this to me?" Why me? Nevertheless, on March 15th at 2:30 in the morning at Sturgeon hospital in St. Albert, Down Syndrome became a reality in our lives.

The night was filled with excitement and anticipation. We were all on edge and full of hope for the end of a perfect pregnancy for my wife, Karen, and the birth of our fourth child. We were hoping for a boy, as we had three wonderful girls. I was anxiously awaiting this birth, with not a thought of the problem that was to ensue. The actual birth was difficult to say the least. With three children already at home and two so close in age, Karen was working full time; she was joyful, but tired. Shawna was our first child and it took us six years to have another. The doctor told us that it was unlikely that we would have any more children, but six years later Jodie came and seventeen months later Paula was born. At this point, the doctor stressed that it would be even more difficult to have another baby, as Karen was not getting any younger.

The pregnancy had been no different than the others preceding it, with a little bleeding in the early part, progressing to a complete nine months without interruptions or any indication that something might be wrong. The labor dragged late into the night. At this point, nothing indicated that there might be any problem with this baby. We had decided to seek the services of a female gynecologist, in accordance with my wife's wishes, and we felt comfortable having her with us. She was prudent, her bedside manner was great and her attitude was remarkable. We felt reassured by her presence and comfortable with her there. As the final preparations were going on, I stood at the head of the bed while Karen was encouraged to push and breathe at regular intervals. The room was dim and quiet. It was getting closer to the time when we would meet our fourth child and fulfill our dream of having a boy. No noise, hospital chatter or nocturnal traffic was evident, as this was the only expected birth in the maternity ward. The only well lit area was immediately in front of the doctor. I felt slightly sick and was happy that the darkness devoured the focus away from me. Karen was tired, but continued her pushing and breathing. The baby was to be larger than our previous three, according to the echo-cardiogram, which reassured me that it would be a healthy baby. The nurses were busy at their task of passing the instruments required for a safe proceeding. All was progressing well, and suddenly the doctor said, "I see the head Karen, just push some more!"

Karen was sleepy, anxious, nervous, and exhausted by her 22 hour labor. I reinforced the doctor's encouragement to Karen, but all she could say was "You caused this, don't tell me to push. I cannot go anymore. If you want, you come and push." I laughed, sympathizing with her. We all chuckled and the doctor exclaimed, "It's a boy, the boy you wanted". As Karen and I hugged and I congratulated her, the doctor, with the nurse, went to the corner of the room and placed the baby in the incubator. Karen wanted to hold our child and I wanted her to have that special moment. After all she did all the work for the miracle which had taken place and she deserved to embrace our son. I looked up and the doctor quietly motioned me over to the far side of the room, which was unlit and suspicious. I was not expecting any problems but the doctor's pensive and inquisitive look shot like a sharp pain through my body. My blood pressure heightened, I held my breath, and wondered what she wanted. I could see the doctor conversing with the nurse and looking perplexed, as she manipulated parts of the baby's body. As I approached, the doctor started to shoot out stats. "The boy is 8 pounds 14 ounces and has brown eyes and brown hair. A rather large size for babies with the condition that I believe your son has." The next part came rather slowly and with a whisper.

"Joe", she said, "I have examined your baby, and I can tell you that with my many years of experience I believe that he has an irreversible condition called Down Syndrome. I am not 100%

certain; we will confirm my diagnosis by performing a Trisomy gene test on the baby. Meanwhile, I have placed him in an incubator; these children often have a series of assorted problems, including bad bowels, intestinal problems, underdeveloped lungs, or an array of heart conditions. As a matter of fact", she explained, "half of all Down syndrome children born have a hole in the heart, congenital in nature. Joe, before we give your son to your wife to hold, what do you want to do? Do you want to tell her now or wait until morning? She is so tired maybe it would be better if we tell her in the morning. That will give her a chance to sleep before having to face the inevitable." I could not think, for through all my professional sports days I had never experienced this kind of pressure, pain and devastation.

I decided, "I think I want to tell her now, I would not want to leave here tonight knowing that Karen was not aware of the condition of our much anticipated baby boy." I thought that I knew my wife best. She would rely on God for help much more then I could, and she would come out better because of her spiritual beliefs. She screamed and looked totally confused when first confronted, but I could sense that a part of her was still composed and, even from the start, ready to take on the challenges of life with and for the son we had both wanted so desperately.

The room quickly cleared of all medical staff, and only one nurse remained to clean up the aftermath of birth and attend to Karen's needs. We were alone. It was at this point that we both realized the enormity of what was ahead of us. Strangely we were not so much worried about our future, as that of our son. We knew nothing of Down Syndrome and less about the problems that the doctor warned could plague our child for life. We both sat there, holding each other, with the same questions and no answers. What is Down Syndrome? What are the implications of the problems associated with it and what could we do? We thought of all the negatives that were to come during the next few days, including informing our friends and relatives who might not understand or care. We both wanted so much for the doctor to be wrong. It has happened before. One of the nurses wheeled Karen back to her room quietly and with no passion. I held her hand and tried not to look at her. All seemed to be well, but not for Karen and me. Our whole world seemed to have caved in on us and in an instant everything had become too difficult to imagine and comprehend. Through out the next morning, the words "Down Syndrome" constantly flashed and regurgitated in my mind.

Depression came over me like a blanket or an unyielding grey curtain. I tried to be of help to Karen, but I was consumed with my own selfish fears about what the next day, next week, next year would bring. Lack of knowledge can be overwhelming and destructive. We had no idea of the nature of the problem, nor how we would or could fulfill our obligation to our child. My instinct was to hate God for if he caused this, then why us? We discussed when it would be best to tell the kids and eventually the family and friends. The family was easy. They would be sleeping therefore to wait until the next morning would be prudent.

I did not want to leave Karen but we decided that I would go home to the kids and be back early the next day. I tried to slip my hand from Karen's grasp, but she was afraid and not willing to let go of my hand. I finally shook from her grasp and headed for the door. As I swung the door open and stepped out into the corridor of the maternity wing, I could hear Karen sobbing in her grief and pain. Tears slowly wound down my cheeks. The emotions of all that had happened overwhelmed me and all that I visualized. I stumbled into the elevator, pressed the button and waited. Usually I find elevators mildly disturbing but this time I was oblivious to the movement and sound. I was engulfed in a dream world, perhaps an automatic reaction of a body system under stress.

The elevator soared to the 4th floor without my notice. I had made a mistake when I pressed the floor number and found myself stepping out into the terrace. I tried to get back in but the emergency door I had stepped out of locked behind me. Lucky for me, a male nurse, out for a smoke, opened the door. I stepped back inside without acknowledging him, but I believe he said hello to me. I got back into the elevator and made sure to press the right button this time. The ride down seemed to slow the night. The noise of the elevator was suppressed and vague. There I was with my solitude, lamenting, but I felt a relief, as I knew that I would meet no one at this point and would not have to explain what happened. I stepped out of the elevator into the lobby.

The lateness of the hour and empty lobby would be my cover. I would not have to reply to any unwelcome questions that soon enough would start for Karen and me. Suddenly a friend of Karen's, a nurse, asked, "Joe how did the delivery go? How is Karen?" I shrugged off her questions. I barely whispered, "fine". In return, she wanted to talk. I showed no willingness. She looked at me and I stared back, shrugged my shoulders and stepped into the brisk March air.

At first I could not find my car or remember in which parking lot I had left it. I recovered my bearings, quickly moved towards my car, and reached into my pocket for the keys. I could not find them. I systematically searched all my pockets over and over, to no avail. Where could they be? Back to the lobby and on to the elevator. I decided to go back to the room in search of the keys. I quietly walked back into Karen's room avoiding all nurses, avoiding lit areas, staying along the wall in the obscurity of the darkness. I slowly swung the door to my wife's room. I was engulfed in the total darkness of the room. I tried desperately to slowly maneuver in the direction of her bed without disturbing her. She was still sobbing. I finally made it to the side of her bed and quietly searched, it seemed in vain, for the keys, on the hospital dresser by her bed. She was in her own world and did not notice as I gently fumbled onto my keys. I turned without disturbing her, slowly found the door and walked out onto the more lit corridor. Back onto the elevator I went, making sure to press the correct button this time. The elevator closed and just as quickly it seemed to open. Back into the chilly night, I finally got to my car. I paused for a minute to digest the situation and consider what I would say to my kids and my family members, remembering that Italian parents and friends would scorn a handicapped child. This was a distorted view, created under severe stress, as my parents and relatives were the salt of the earth, and furthest from what I imaged. I turned the ignition and pressed on the gas. The car rolled slowly out of the parking lot and onto the icy streets. It did not matter; it seemed nothing mattered. There was nothing I could think of or dream of that would make this night go away. My thoughts went back to my kids, to what I would say to them. How would they react? How could I say it to shield them from the reality of this night?

As I drove closer and closer to my street, I envisioned that perhaps it was a dream; yes a dream, it could be a dream. My imagination was racing and it felt so good to step out of reality for just a while. As I turned into my driveway, all the lights were off. Great, I thought, they are all asleep. If they were, I could wait till morning to inform them of what happened. I made certain not to slam the car door, to avoid awakening anyone in the house. I opened the side door and climbed two stairs leading to the kitchen, refraining from turning on the lights. I stepped slowly and quietly down the hall towards my room, hoping not to attract attention.

Suddenly I was met by screaming lights coming from all the girls' rooms. Shawn, Jodie, and Paula had all anticipated my arrival and were anxiously and excitedly awaiting the news. How did it go Dad?" Exclaimed Shawna. "Was it a boy or a girl?"

Without giving all the details, I told them that there were some complications and the doctor thought that perhaps the baby has Downs. But we were not certain, until this Trisomy 21 test, which I had never heard of previously. This particular test however cannot be performed at the present hospital. "Don't worry girls, all will be fine. Tomorrow we will all go see your mom and all will be fine." What time can we go?" they insisted. I reminded them that they had school in the morning and that after that I would take them to the hospital to see her. I also explained that the baby would have to be transported to the University of Alberta hospital and Mom would come home alone. They persisted, "What is the problem? What is Downs?" I cut the questions off and told them that all would be fine. "Let's all go to bed. We will talk in the morning". Reluctant, and perhaps feeling much as their mother and I felt when the news was given to us, they had many more questions. But there would be no answers this night. There was nothing I could say that would pacify or reassure them. So I did not attempt what seemed impossible for them to comprehend.

Shawna was courageous and a real trooper. She reassured her sisters, told them to go to bed; all would be fine. She even attempted to reassure me. My kids were stronger than I had anticipated, and more calm and pragmatic than I. We all went to bed. It was 4:00a.m. and the sun would be up soon. I did not want morning to come; I closed my eyes and wished that all would be as it was prior to the birth. I tried in vain to think of all positives that could eventually take place. But I could not come up with any. I decided that at this point it would not be wise to continue in this line of thought but instead I would plan my action for the morning: go to the hospital; console my wife and daughters; and start the process of reading all I could and learning all I could on the subject.

The morning came; signs of spring were creeping in. The sun was piercing through the curtains showing signs of warming the veil of winter away. Spring came earlier than anticipated. Birds chirped on the rooftops, the noise of our crescent awakening to the fresh morning air. The sounds of garage and car doors echoed in the wind, neighbours leaving the comfort of their homes and making their way to their daily work, or other destinations. It all seemed so placid, so bright, and so routine, but I felt alone in my solitude and anguish.

I knew that Karen would be feeling the same, perhaps worse, as she too would face this morning much like me, desolate and alone. I knew I needed to be there to hold her hand and console her as she awakened into the reality of our new situation. I quickly dashed out of bed and into the shower. I could not concentrate on what clothing to wear, which shirt with which pants, but it did not seem to matter. I found myself in the car without concern for any of the daily hygiene. The car was cold and windows needed scraping from the night frost. I scratched a hole in the center of the windshield on the driver's side and quickly started the car. Backing up without looking, I almost hit the next door neighbour.

I slammed the car into forward gear and dashed for the hospital. It took me very little time to get there; it was all just a blur. When I arrived, the parking lot was just starting to awaken and the admitting section was busy. I parked without taking a parking ticket and made a mad rush for the elevator. Once in the elevator, I remembered not to repeat the mistake of the night before, and correctly pressed the third floor button. As the elevator reached the third floor, and the door swung open, I noticed that they were wheeling Karen into her room. They had obviously taken her for some early testing. I quickly dashed into her room and approached her bed.

A nurse was organizing her drip and maneuvering her sheets and blankets. The nurse reacted to my approach with a cautious smile. She then told Karen and me that our life with Josh would be difficult at best and many things would probably go wrong. As she continued to fabricate a litany of wrongs-to-be, Karen and I, for the first time, really listened. What we heard was a chorus of negatives. Not one positive note from any nurse, doctor, or hospital administrator since Karen had given birth to Josh. I did not fault them, for that time in history their reasoning was sound. We soon realized, as we embarked on our journey down the next few days and continued to hear from many other hospital officials, that we would hear not one consoling or hopeful insight about the future of our boy and his chances for a normal and productive life. It struck me as odd that there could be nothing positive about a child's birth, that in history nothing had developed, that these kids, with this affliction could not be validated as being good or positive.

At this point Karen and I conferred, and realized that we needed to take our lives, and that of our boy, into our hands. We were determined to make a positive future for him and for us. It would be difficult, almost impossible, as we had no medical knowledge, nor previous personal experience, but we were prepared to try. We both started to listen more closely to everyone who spoke for or against our child and his condition. From that point we

10

immediately started to read all that we could--any book, any research, any film on his condition, any minute scrap of information we could devour and learn would help.

The social worker, in the presence of a doctor, would once again confirm that we had an option to take Josh home, take care of him and love him, or do what over fifty percent of other parents who have children with a multitude of defects do: leave him in the hospital, in the hands of the government, and make him a ward of the state. Both Karen and I sat there, mentally, and somewhat physically, paralyzed at that statement.

I replied, "What? What did you say? Did I hear you correctly? Karen, did I hear her correctly?" Karen could give no answer, just a disgusted stare into space. It seems that I had heard this before but never did it register. This time it was staring at both of us and it was clear that they wanted an answer. "Think about it", the social worker went on, "and give us an answer. You have a short time to decide. You are ready to take the baby home today, and an immense amount of paper work is required should you choose to leave him with the state." I was inclined to make judgment on those who leave their mentally or physically handicapped children behind; however I could not. We all have explainable reasons for our actions. Those who chose that course in the past, or do so today, have to deal with their own consciences. I knew that I would regret it had I made that decision. It was time to take Josh home. All that could be done had been done. We were on our own now. I gathered all of Karen's belongings, while she cared for Josh. Best wishes came from all the medical staff and the staff of the hospital's neonatal clinic. Their kind words were appreciated but not heard, nor did they penetrate our souls. Ultimately it would be up to us.

Down the elevator and to the parking lot, we had no problem finding the car. The flowers, we left behind. They reminded us of our solitude to come. Karen held Josh. She refused to let him go, and refused to talk about any of the issues. As we pulled out of the parking lot and onto the street, the morning air was biting but inviting. The sun was up and smiling on us through the windows; we basked in it; it seemed so reassuring. We drove for home and nothing was said, each of us caught in our own thoughts. Our minds swam in waves of doubt and fear, fear for the future and doubt as to how we would handle it.

Tears came to my eyes at the thought of what could have been. As an athlete and a coach I envisioned a son whom I could work with and mold into a great athlete, and have him accomplish all those things that eluded me in my sports experience, and correct all those sports mistakes I had foolishly made. I took for granted that my son would be the vehicle which would allow me to vicariously live the reality of a proud father and share with him all my experiences. I would have tried to imagine Josh as a Special Olympic athlete, had I any idea what it was, where to turn, or if such a thing existed. A strange world had beset us and we knew nothing about it. Much had to be studied and learned, from the sports he could play, the schools he could attend, the doctors, other agencies we could frequent, the books to read, the movies to watch, the clinics available. The knowledge required to take on the job of making Josh a life and allowing him to live it seemed immeasurable.

As I drove, I didn't know what was occupying Karen's thoughts, but I did know her. She is much more trusting of God and faith-filled. She would wish nothing for herself and all for Josh, and would give herself in totality for the betterment of our son. She would make certain that Josh received the best education, the best books, the best clothing and all the support needed to stimulate his environment and make a better place for him. While I had selfishly been thinking more of how Josh's birth would affect me and all those around us, I knew that Karen's vision would always be how to ensure that everything around Josh would affect him in a positive way. My wife, even on that day, was ready to implement all that she would learn on the benefits of stimulation, sound integrated schools, genuine teachers, heart warming teacher assistants, and accepting care givers, such as herself, and start a new chapter in the world of Down Syndrome, and of Josh.

She would, in her own way, illuminate the way for Josh so that he could grow to his God-given potential, surrounded by loving family and friends. She was certain of the outcome. I wasn't so certain of anything at that point. Little did I realize that Josh would transcend all hates, mold and inspire our love for each other, kindle our hearts, bring togetherness to our family, cure all depression with his smile and illuminating eyes, love unconditionally, and hate but for one minute at most. I cannot now imagine our family without him. The journey began that day when we made that pledge to Josh, when we decided that we would not dwell in the negative, but accentuate and immerse ourselves in the positive and in all we could bring to Josh.

JOSH'S HUMOR

I have spent much time with a very close friend lately, as we are presently attempting to deliver his very athletic son to a European team for a position on their soccer roster and eventually a signing of a major contract. He phones me often, and on many occasions, Josh answers the phone. Josh, who is witty if not sarcastic, answered the phone one night and when my friend asked for me, Josh replied "Just a minute, I will get him". He then called in a loud tone," Dad, It's your boyfriend on the line." Stella, Carmelo's wife, who heard the yell laughed hysterically as I made my way to the phone. When we get together with Carmelo and his family, this event is often repeated.

CHAPTER
2

The Home Life

As days went by, I read as many books as possible while Karen researched the Down's community for any or all available resources. As we continued to ponder our next moves to meet Josh's specific needs, we realized that a tiny, yes, very tiny, light was visible at the end of a rather large tunnel. The dreariness and gloom portrayed by all we had encountered could be combated. Karen and I decided that we would take this journey together, along with our kids, and make Josh's life as enriching, exciting, positive, stimulating, and lasting as possible. It would not be easy, but our effort, all of our family's efforts and that of our friends, and our love and devotion would prevail. We settled in our home and after the initial worries and concerns, new ones erupted: we worried about everything from what to feed Josh, how to feed him, which bed to place him in, which blankets to use, and how much stimulation would be needed.

A schedule was devised so that Josh would receive stimulation for all his five senses at all times. Unlike the early days of all our other children, we were all preoccupied with every minute detail concerning Josh.--perhaps too much. The colour in his room, the games he would play or we would play for him or with him; the music he would listen to, everything became crucial. We were destined to compensate and overwork on all fronts relating to the wellbeing of our boy. He would beat the odds and live as healthy a life as possible. We wanted to develop and perhaps invent something new with Down's and defy the odds. Talking, reading, singing, manipulating his arms and legs, strengthening his neck muscles and stomach muscles: stimulation and activity were continual, tedious and fastidious.

As it took much longer for him to swallow food, he could not be breastfed. He still had to be trained to suck on the bottle nipples and then ingest the food, however. Swallowing, while seemingly a natural response, is not natural for babies with Down's. He had to be continually conditioned. He lacked strength in his jaws and mouth, and the length of time it took to eat would usually be doubled. It seemed that we would go from one feeding to the next, as it took so long on each occasion. We also fretted about the possibility of aspiration pneumonia setting in if he ingested food down the wrong pipe. It was during these first days and months that we came to realize that everything Josh would achieve would come down to repetition and stimulation in specific aspects of all tasks.

For too long, people had believed that nothing could be done for those afflicted by this congenital disease. Therefore Down's children were placed in mental hospitals, destined to spend the rest of their lives there. This validated people's idea that Down's children could not be taught. Today the general consensus is that with care, stimulation, early intervention, and continual work on the mental and physical growth of these children, tremendous results are possible. Josh is a proof of positive effects of constant stimulation, both on a physical and mental level, on these children.

We have found that with stimulation and devotion to all aspects of their development, these children can challenge their "destiny". With integrated classes, integrated in a public school system, and with participation in as many community activities as possible, these children can learn to read, write, and cope with most of the daily social skills required for life in our society. School integration also helps to bridge the gap with kids who are not afflicted with Down's, and helps them to learn how to interact with children with disabilities. In fact I believe that integration has and will continue to allow Josh to be a productive member of our society. Karen and I are not naïve. We know that while integration is great up to a certain point; total integration is neither possible nor is it a benefit to Josh. A well-balanced, integrated program along with individualized attention can be extremely beneficial to the Down's child.

Days went by, weeks and months. We were all busy being a normal family while still giving just a little more for Josh. Our other kids were wonderful in every way. They would take turns with chores, cooking, baby sitting and cleaning up after Josh. Josh and Megan were assigned to our official babysitter, who babysat all of our kids, a good-hearted person, caring and easy going with the children. My life as usual was much easier, as I continued to teach and coach, keeping myself busy to avoid continual thinking. Karen was the real center of our family universe, of all that went on and is going on with the family. It was, and still is, Karen on whom all of us rely for encouragement and comforting.

Josh crawled quickly but walked much later. Down's children have a condition that affects their muscles, which makes them floppy, soft and stretchy. His jaw muscles and neck muscles were weaker. His stomach muscles were floppy and easily stretched, so he looked like he had a "beer gut".

The feet of children with Down Syndrome are usually flat, and their hands are stubby and the palms show an imprint of their genetic malfunction. Their noses are slightly turned up, their ears are usually smaller and indented. Their eyes, oval in shape, are like those of a Mongol; thus the condition's original name "mongoloid". This term is no longer used and the official name for the medical condition is Down Syndrome. Their chins are shorter and their necks more compressed. Their tongues are slightly larger than the size of their mouth, as the mouth is less developed. This puts the tongue in a protruding position because it does not fit completely within the mouth. Because of this, Down Syndrome children find it more difficult to chew and swallow food. During their first few years these children need to be watched at all times when they eat. They need to be reminded constantly about the virtues of eating more slowly and chewing less and more often. On three different occasions I had to perform the Heimlich Maneuver on Josh as he has repeatedly ingested more food than he could chew on all occasions. We have been very fortunate; however, things only have to go bad one time. The last time it happened, we were, to begin with, many miles away from an emergency room and had things gone badly, it would have been disastrous.

During supper one weekend at the lake, Josh placed on his plate an enormous amount of food, as Down's children like to do. He took two or three pork ribs that were boned and rather large. I border on paranoia when he eats, as I have been the one who has had to perform the critical maneuvers on all of these occasions. As I watched him attack the ribs, I sensed that something was about to ensue. When he placed the rib into his mouth and closed it, I realized that he had it all inside of his mouth. His mouth remained closed and he persisted in chewing the meat portion of the bone. As I looked again it seemed he was gasping for air, yet he was not making any gestures of panic or needing help.

He continued to sit immobilized but showed no signs of wanting help. I got out of my chair, some distance away on a rather large patio. As I approached to investigate, I noticed that he was not able to breathe as he was definitely gasping for air. I also realized that his mouth no longer seemed full and enlarged as it had previously. When I drew closer yet, he signaled to his throat and sat there dispassionately, almost with confidence that I would come to his rescue as I had previously. In a panic I got behind him and crossed my arms and locked them into place in front of his diaphragm, just below the sternum bone. As I started to press inward and upward towards his throat, I remembered from the previous two times that the spot might not be contacted the first time, therefore, many maneuvers in slightly different areas of the upper stomach area would have to be primed. It must be stressed at this time that the magic spot may not be contacted, in which case 911 would have to be called.

On I went, and it seemed forever. I called for Karen to get ready to call 911 should I not be successful. Many seconds had lapsed, as I continued to press, hoping to hit that magic spot which would automatically project the food outward, as I had been blessed to see on previous occasions. Time was ticking. I had asked Karen to count the seconds for me. Thirty seconds went by as I became more frantic to accomplish what seemed impossible. Harder and harder I pressed, each time hoping for a miracle. Forty seconds and no positive result. I started to contemplate a possible tracheotomy as a last resort. But this would mean having to cut down his windpipe and place a circular tube of any sort down his throat. Having only read about it and having never performed it, the outcome could be scary at best.

Sixty seconds: it seemed forever. I continued to probe at slightly different angles, hoping, praying and then suddenly, as I made my next drastic maneuver, a full boned rib at least five inches in length ejected like a projectile from his mouth and his slightly bluish face slowly regained its normal colour with every panicked breath he took. The salvation of the day had to be first all of the prayers, and secondly the fact that the ribs contained a good amount of oil and moisture, which allowed the bone to dislodge from the throat and up onto the grass. I cannot stress enough from our personal experiences, the need to teach Down's children--to remind them at every meal--to chew more and slowly. Because of my diligence, Josh refuses to sit by me at the supper table, knowing full well that I will be on his case; however, it's worth it. The Down's sternum bone is less defined and late in developing, creating a fossa within, in early years. Their heads are slightly bigger than other parts of the body, per proportion to size at birth.

The metabolism of a Down Syndrome child is more passive than normal; therefore these kids will always overeat, and if not watched carefully, will continually indulge in food or drink. Because his brain takes longer to notify the rest of the body (mostly the stomach) that it is satiated and ready to stop intake of food, we have had a major problem with Josh in this regard. We have tried every remedy with very little success and our concern is that if continued into his adult years, he will without a doubt develop physical problems as a result. We did try to lock all the food areas around the house, and we placed a lock on the fridge itself. This was successful but we were not able to justify the method. We had to find another way. We started to stress the concept of eating healthy for a better life, and explained to Josh the consequences of poor eating habits. We now collectively ensure that whoever is eating with Josh will always get him to eat smart and healthy.

He has bought into the plan and he now only eats food from places like Subway where he receives portions that are large enough to satisfy him but healthy enough to satisfy us. Although Josh participates in many activities, he has gained weight, mostly in his stomach area. We are working on a fitness program for Josh, and his sisters have bought a pass at the fitness center. He faithfully goes when they go and takes part in a semi-rigorous activity plan aside from all his other sport activities. This has helped him to lower his weight and gain more muscle tone and strength.

Some Down's children are born with a slight asthmatic condition. Josh has some difficulty with this. Moreover, because they are more flexible and their muscles stretch and give more, all are physically, not just mentally and emotionally delayed, depending on the severity of the congenital problem at the moment of conception.

Because of their lax muscle structure these kids experience physical developmental delays. We constantly evaluated, measured, weighed, looked, stretched, lifted, and grabbed all parts of his body, questioned all that we saw or, mostly, thought we saw. Even his bowel movements, which were slightly retarded but within parameters of normal kids, were scrutinized. His walking was slightly slowed but not too profoundly. A rather large baby in weight and size for Downs, we noticed no other physical defects. As for his cognitive development, we desperately contrived proven and unproven methodology for a brighter, stronger child.

Every step of the way, we measured his results against the "norms" and either sobbed or rejoiced at each of the results. It is natural that we would do that, and while we negated any importance was attached to our testing and documentation, we were nevertheless consumed by his results or lack thereof at every instance. Any positive thing that he did was always a discussion for every family meeting or get together. We would share all that transpired with Josh with everyone to prove his normalcy. Perhaps, we, as all parents and relatives of kids with birth defects, do tend to bypass the negative and accentuate any small, even tiny, positive, so that we can go on and feel good about what we are doing. We frequented numerous households with babies such as ours and took advantage of their past experiences. We attended encounter meetings with other couples who had given birth to children with disabilities. Basically, we were consumed by, and grasped at, the elusive fountain of hope for ourselves and Josh.

JOSH'S HUMOR

One night on the way home from Tuesday night floor hockey, I asked Josh, with no thought as to his response, what he would do if I died suddenly, reminding him that he would be the man of the house and he would have to take over all my responsibilities. He had two quick answers. First, he exclaimed, "Party time!" Second, he gasped, "No, no you mean I have to sleep with my mother?" This is the spontaneity and wit that Josh exhibits on many occasions and every moment spent with him is truly constant laughter and a heart-warming experience. Now that I spend more time with Josh due to my reduced involvement with soccer and teaching, I am fascinated by his exuberance and enthusiasm for everything, every day. On many occasions people with whom we come in contact, who have never before experienced or known Josh, people in malls, stores, schools and other public places, will give Josh products at half price if not for free. We want to pay but they insist on a gesture of love for a special child. One day Josh was in line with his mother, at a cashier in Sobeys grocery store, when the cashier noticed that Josh had picked up a two liter bottle of coke and was ready to open his wallet to pay. She told him to keep the money and that the coke was "on her". Karen, realizing what had happened, thanked the lady and suggested that she would pay. The lady replied, "I don't go to church; this is my small deed of sharing with an innocent boy who God has placed on this earth to remind us all of our daily duty to help those in our community who need it."

CHAPTER
3

The Early Years

When Josh started pre-school the situation and the habits, for us, all were the same. We continued to fret, and now we were concerned with his reaction to other children and theirs to him, as well as the reaction of the caregivers, for whom every little situation would create a crisis. From the first day of school, through no one's fault, we were faced with the appropriateness of Josh's actions in all situations. Josh pulled the fire alarm, causing a disturbance and a small crisis for the school, especially considering that it was -40 centigrade. Josh did not leave the school in a panic as all the other kids, teachers and administrators were forced to; rather Josh calmly put on his coat, hat and boots and then stepped outside knowing full well that all was fine.

This became a crisis that, according to those few teachers, who hated integration, could not be tolerated. According to them, it was only because Josh was Down's that it happened. I tried to explain to the staff that I teach in high school and we have at least two fire alarm pulls per year committed by "normal" and in many cases very high I.Q. kids. However, some teachers felt that while "normal" kids will do stupid things and should be excused, what Josh did should not be tolerated because it was a stupid person doing the act. For the normal kid, a prank; for Josh, a mentally retarded episode, by a boy who is mentally retarded. We had to fight against this kind of stupidity on many fronts, and on many occasions. At this point, I don't want to lay blame, for Downs do things which not only appear abnormal, but are, in fact, abnormal, because that's precisely what they are. Despite the difficulties his actions may cause, our boy has provided us with countless stories and moments of laughter.

Most stories are funny and a few are funny but dangerous. With Josh, we have learned that you must be vigilant, for he is likely to act or react to situations and at times danger can be created; however, with hard work, the mental capacity of Down's can in most cases be increased. When you explain to Josh a social or life skill, he understands the immediate concept rather well; however, he is not cognizant of all the peripheral common sense branches within every situation. If you tell Josh that in some situation he is not to turn left because a car will come and hit him, he does not connect this to the fact that if he turns right he can also get run over. Therefore he must also be told that the second option is also important.

Because there are many variations to all social and life skills, and because Josh learns by continual repetitions, attention must be paid to all side stories or the teachings of every story. For example, we have four daughters and Josh is exposed by visualization and stimulated by all that he sees them do. He may not connect to the specific situation and may apply his observations to other applications and this could result in problems for him. One day Josh found his sisters' tampons – Because they are long, thin and white, he assumed that they could be smoked as cigarettes and one day he brought a whole case to school. This was in grade three. He then went on and passed them out to every child in the class as cigarettes. All of the children took one and were pretending to smoke them.

The teacher was outraged that Josh would do that and implied, that only a mentally challenged person could think of that. What she did not take into account of course, was that all the kids in Josh's class, were using them as cigarettes. These children are spontaneous and react to all situations with vivid and explicit imaginations.

Just when you think he has not caught onto a conversation, you find that he has absorbed all that he hears, but not necessarily understood the intent of the story. Our girls took an interest in him, whenever they returned from school or from being out with their friends. On many occasions, the girls would bring back friends after their dates or outings, and everyone enjoyed Josh immensely. Their interactions with Josh helped the development of Josh's social skills. Josh was involved with every aspect of his sisters' lives and our family in general. He was taken to every one of their sports events and he seemed to look forward to all the soccer games, basketball games, and other activities in which the girls participated. This allowed him to learn at an early age to deal with outside influences and socializing outside the family circle.

Because the first three years of upbringing were mostly home related, some of his abnormal behavior was tolerated and rather enjoyed. His mental handicaps were funny and rather unique. Indirectly, all of us dreaded the day when Josh would be less protected and in an environment in which he might not be able to cope. I was especially concerned with his first day at school and the reaction of his teachers, peers, and their parents, to his physical appearance and slight mental deviation. Josh was enrolled in integrated schools from preschool, on. The preschool was a non-denominational school in the Protestant tradition.

We also soon learned that those children who were swayed towards some form of repulsion for Josh, had been influenced by the reactions of the parents, who were full of resentment for Josh's being in the same class with their sons or daughters. Their contention was that having Josh amongst them would slow the progress that their child could make. They were appalled and slightly irritated if the teacher gave more attention to Josh and his needs, believing this to be detrimental to their child. I can respect that attitude, while seeing it as totally misguided on their part; but I was looking at the situation from the perspective of the benefits to Josh, without rendering a glance at what this could or would do for the other students.

Josh did progress and learn at a slower pace than the other children, but at a fast pace for his capacity. We realized later, that those kids who had entered preschool, would eventually continue with Josh in his future formative school years develop an engaging and ever growing fraternity with, and love for him. Integration did work and it has worked for Josh. For the second year, we kept Josh back in preschool for one more year as Megan (our fourth and youngest daughter) was entering preschool and it would be great if she could help Josh along. We also felt that it would give Josh more time to mature prior to kindergarten. We weren't certain how Megan would react or face the challenge of having her handicapped brother in the same class. She had never been placed in a position where she would have to deal with the outside world, and Josh, in the same room, every day. Once again our fears were groundless. Megan seemed to take her responsibility with grace and in a more mature way than I might have.

As his father, I fretted and dreaded every day that exposed Josh to the potential of laughter and ridicule from the outside world. I always was more sensitive to people's reaction to Josh (in part due to my Italian upbringing) than the rest of the family seemed to be. While I loved and always will love Josh, I, more than Karen and the kids, seemed unnerved at all the public response to Josh. Because of Megan's influence, this included a positive and caring affection for her brother. I never heard her complain or express disgust at any of the daily events at play-school. She seemed distant to adverse reactions on a daily basis. I knew then that Megan would remain a great role model and caring influence for Josh in the years to come.

Can't Hold Me Down   Joe Petrone

JOSH'S HUMOR

One day the principal called and told us that Josh had been disrespectful to one of his teachers. We were somewhat surprised and wanted to put a quick stop to that sort of action. We wanted to be forceful in our approach with him when he got home. As he stepped into the house, he realized that we would confront him eventually; therefore, he walked up to us both and demanded punishment for his actions immediately.

We proceeded to give him a firebrand reason for not repeating his action. When we were both finished our outburst, we paused and Karen asked him why he swore at the teacher. His reply? "I'm handicapped; what do you expect?" We found it difficult not to smile at his answer, and sternly repeated our disgust for his actions. We realized moreover that his answer was sincere and truthfully given. He was not being sarcastic, but merely reiterating the perception of who he was and was constantly told he was. We had no answer, for on many occasions we all had referred to him as "handicapped."

CHAPTER
4

Kindergarten

For kindergarten, Josh joined Megan at a new school. This, like all new experiences, would be a challenge for Josh, and us, as new situations always led to apprehensions. One consolation was that Megan could be trusted to be with Josh, support him, and continue to indirectly attend to his needs. She also had to remain in the background and not personally get involved in every situation that arose and cause an overprotective barrier for Josh with teachers, administration, and other kids.

The reality of Josh's growth in size and mental capacity would be a continual challenge. His ability to develop at or close to normal range would be tested every day and immediately evaluated by us. The rest of the kids would be the gauge of his progression, by their response to him on a daily basis. We were told that as Josh increased in age and maturity, he would get further and further behind physically and mentally with respect to other kids. This left us with a frightening vision of the implications for his future.

Orientation went well. All of the other children and their parents were introduced at the first meeting, as were we and Josh, and were evaluated by other parents. Most parents were not aware that Josh would be part of the class. Again, the kids never noticed, but all the parents asked a few honest and reasonable questions pertaining to Josh and their child's development in an integrated class. Josh's teacher assistant was introduced and everyone was made aware that Josh would take part in all class activities, with some individualized days for him with the assistant. The teacher reassured the parents that Josh's being there would not in any way take away from their children's social, physical, or cognitive growth. The parents were also told that a new program of integration would be the future order of the day, as the Provincial Department of Education had decreed that all classrooms in Alberta would be integrated. It did slightly unnerve and cause discomfort to some parents, but all were prepared to be open minded and give Josh and other special children a fighting chance, as close as possible to a normal experience in life.

The order of the day, as Josh started his educational climb was integrated, interceptive stimulation. The model school would have all kids with special needs in this new innovative program, which was designed to save money for the community and the educational system, and enrich the educational experience of the disabled child. Most, but not all teachers were neither affirmative of nor congenial to the program, for it created many hardships. The concern of educators, who were in the "trenches" on a day-to-day basis, overseeing and attempting to teach in already overcrowded classes with little or no support in order to meet what they would definitely consider a supreme challenge, was warranted. There were two choices with which a parent of both the special needs child and the normal child would be faced: to go along and embrace the future, or fight it and endanger not only the future of special kids but also the educational, mental and physical development of "normal" children involved in this integrated system.

Karen, our kids, and I, embraced the idea of change and desperately ran with it. Everything that Josh was involved with at school, my wife and kids became a part of. They offered to read to the students, play with the kids, and work with the teachers and staff at every turn, anything to help when they could, for the betterment of all the children and eventually Josh. I was, to a lesser degree, doing the same. Together our family spent countless hours, days, and months assisting, and in some case leading and driving, with integrated intervention with a certain amount of stimulative fervor, as to satisfy every need for the teacher, all for Josh's benefit.

Josh worked with "normal" children every day and after school hours we compensated by placing him in an overwhelming number of selected, stimulating activities. Josh played in an organized and structured soccer program; we also enrolled him in a music program where he studied the piano. It is fitting that Josh seemed to have the same intuition about piano lessons as my other kids, who all took piano for years. He hated and dreaded each and every piano lesson he took; just like my other children (and a great majority of all the children who are in piano lessons). His disdain for piano was not the fault of the teacher, who was a wonderful mentor for Josh and all my kids.

One day Karen told me that the piano teacher would have to stop teaching as her breast cancer had reoccurred and she was given but a few months to live. On the last day of classes I drove Josh to piano lessons as always, but on this day I had to tell him that Mrs. Stanton was dying and that this particular lesson would be his last.

I wasn't certain how to break the news to Josh, or whether to tell him prior to or after the last session. I decided to wait until the lesson was over. When I picked him up and he got into the car, I explained to him that he could not go to piano anymore as Mrs. Stanton was dying. Without hesitation he replied, "There is a God up there; I hate piano." Josh really loved Mrs. Stanton and she was very fond of him, but Josh could not connect that her dying was completely connected to his stoppage of piano lessons. He did cry at her funeral but once again it was in a different context. Later we enrolled Josh in dancing in the hope that music would stimulate and invigorate his mind, while also help to develop balance and grace.

Part of the integration aspect of the school that Josh attended was to assimilate children with special needs into student life as much as possible. The drama teacher at the school was a wonderfully gifted lady, not only in acting and drama, but also in showing love and support for Josh. She allowed Josh to be integrated in the year play and a special part for him was created. Josh's participation completely quieted any rumblings about the ability of these kids to learn. From Grades 1 to 6 Josh's disabilities were not as visible.
He did all things academically, physically, and emotionally, in the same range as the normal children and to a lesser degree; even with those more gifted ones. Josh could read somewhat as well, and write as well as most could then, and his learning curve only slightly lagged behind other students. In athletics he surpassed many of the other students and was equal to those in the top range of skill level. He danced with the best, was inquisitive, continually did his homework, and asked questions in class. He had an instinct for theatrics and from day to day came up with more than his share of creative, though somewhat disruptive ideas.

One morning Josh walked to school, which was rare for him. It had rained for days and rain was still coming down softly this particular morning. As Josh slowly walked towards the school he noticed a multitude of worms swiveling along the sidewalks. Josh came up with the idea that he would pick them up and take them to school so the teacher could use them to teach a science lesson. It was very imaginative of him, but he had no place to put them and nothing in which to carry them. He decided to put them in his pockets. He gathered over fifty of them and happily walked into school, eager to show his teacher his accomplishment. He really believed that giving them to his teacher was a stroke of kindness and caring. Of course, he had no way of knowing that his teacher had a phobia of worms. He called to her as he approached, and then excitedly emptied his pockets full of worms onto her desk. She gasped and screamed from fright. Unable to even ask him to take them away, she watched in horror as the worms over took her desk and slowly maneuvered their way onto her lesson plans. Unable to bear another second, she ran out of the class, leaving Josh confused and perplexed. Hearing the screaming and commotion, another teacher walked into the room. Once she saw why her colleague had run from the room, she, too, refused to enter. Finally, another student came to the rescue, and with Josh's help grabbed the worms and placed them outside. Josh never could understand the reaction from the teachers, as he thought he had done a good deed. It is the lack of peripheral understanding which these kids face every day.

Like other special kids, Josh often makes decisions based on good intentions, but which in fact can cause many problems, especially without a vigilant eye. Josh has always wanted independence, and feels that he is an individual who should be allowed to make his own choices. As his parents, we must allow him to feel independent and assert himself, while at the same time maintaining constant vigilance. Down's children can never be totally self sufficient and can never be placed in a position where they are on their own for a long period of time, such as weeks or months. Many parents may hope this can be, but it will never actually happen. Unfortunately, because of this, a majority of these kids are abandoned and placed in the hands of the government. This results in these kids being placed in group homes with some guidance from social workers, but in many cases left on their own. Moreover, the amount of money that these kids receive from the government every month is so unsatisfactory they often face severe hardship.

One aspect of Josh's personality was his lack of fear or inhibition in front of an audience. He thrived on it, loved it, cherished it, and had an aptitude for acting, dancing, singing, and making a "ham bone" out of himself. Josh and Down's kids are dare devils and will attempt absolutely any stunt which they are shown, without fear of any sort. For example, Josh, like all the other students in his grade 6 class, took a trip to the mountains to ski for two days as part of their physical education class. Josh had never skied before. As a beginner, he had to spend time with the instructor to learn how to get all the equipment on, as well as the basic elements of skiing. Most of his classmates had never been on skis before either. Once the instructor finished the thirty minute lesson, he asked all the students to get ready to "snow plow" down the hill. Josh turned to face the course and without hesitation ripped down the hill at maximum speed. He continued at that pace without ever slowing down. When he finally ran into the line of skiers who were ready to go up the towline, he had literally plowed close to thirty bystanders; he of course got up, laughed, and got ready to go back up, unaware of the danger in which he had placed himself and others.

JOSH'S HUMOR

A teacher's assistant who spent many days and months with Josh, bears witness to the fact that Josh had no enemies, only friends. He had no hate for anyone and enjoyed people from all walks of life, of all colors and ethnic ties. Once day he was asked by Mrs. Hooper to create a pictorial collage of family members, relatives, friends and caregivers with whom he had a special bond. In his collage he placed a picture of a black boy whom he had met but once.

Mrs. Hooper asked him why he ha had placed a picture of a boy he hardly knew with those of his family and friends. Josh replied, "He was nice to me; he played with me, smiled at me and cared. I like him. I think I would like to invite him to my house for supper one evening." And he did just that; he invited him for one of our Sunday suppers, where we met a talkative, gracious, happy boy who seemed to enjoy all of our company. The boy has since reciprocated and asked Josh to go to his house for a meal.   He is now a good friend and close to Josh.

CHAPTER
5

Elementary/Junior High Years

When Josh was in elementary school, we quickly recognized that he had many extraordinary traits. In competitive sports, Josh could perform better than most. Due to the care taken by my son-in law (Chris), Josh could absorb skills and perform. My son-in law spent hours in the backyard with Josh, working on different sports and on the different skills required. Josh is especially suited, gifted at baseball. He spent many days out in the yard learning from Chris. He also spends days in front of the television absorbing every move of his favorite team, the Toronto Blue Jays. He imitated the idiosyncrasies of the sport, and the athletes, and adapted them all within his own game in Special Olympics baseball.

He was also a superb floor hockey player, and thanks to Chris, who is a former AAA midget hockey player and presently the coach for the Merchants Junior hockey team, Josh has been able to develop an understanding for the game and is equipped with the best shot in the league, scoring many goals and finding satisfaction in the sport and his teammates. He, like all athletes, is very much aware of his natural skills and is not afraid to capitalize on any and all accolades that are thrown his way. A superb hitter, Josh led his special Olympic baseball team to many tournaments, and accumulated many home runs.

Everything Josh does is done with gusto and care. While I did spend time on his football and soccer skills, as that is my strength, he has not taken to those sports with the vigor of the others. He enjoyed all activities and thrived at the response from his family, friends and fellow players. Josh particularly enjoyed the post-scoring extravaganza that he learned from watching the antics of those players playing in World Cup Soccer. He also imitated the Italian first division and the now-defunct Drillers of the indoor league, by taking off his shirt and blowing kisses. With every goal he scored, he ran along the sidelines engaging in high fives with all his teammates.

Initially we were told, and continually reminded, of the many difficulties we would experience in our lives because of Josh's birth. It was even suggested that we leave him as a ward of the government. Perhaps there are those people who have kept their mentally and physically handicapped child and things have not gone so well. Nothing ever goes according to plan. Nothing ever goes perfectly well in life. What you and I make of life is the sweat and tears that we all devote to that God-given life.

Today, the reality is that many kids who are, or we claim are, "normal" actually suffer from laziness, lack of respect for their family and friends, and disgust for teachers, their community, the law, and the court system. While most of the kids I teach in high school are superb young individuals, a few achieve much less than

Josh, for they waste their God-given talents by skipping classes, or by taking or selling drugs. These kids are often unable, or unwilling to attend classes are often high, and usually totally ineffective. They live in a world of superficial commercialism and are usually the bullies of the school. These are the kids who are bored with school and find themselves in peril with the law. These are the children of parents who decided to have kids but did not face the responsibility of raising them. The parents of these kids, who are part of the "me" generation, place themselves ahead of the betterment of their kids and produce those kids who on a daily basis are questioned by school administrators or the police.

Our administrators devote 95% of their time to the same twenty kids, while having to neglect the rest. Every year billions of dollars are spent by educational systems and our criminal justice in the pursuit and containment of these individuals, in all schools, in every city and town in this country. These billions would be better spent on all those people who work to their potential, Special needs kids are doing their best while suffering from physical and mental pain, and their faces tell the story. Watch them, should they score a goal, win a race, read a book or learn to write. They care and want to learn all that is within their ability. They enjoy all they do and treasure every moment. With our care and love, Special Olympic kids will be solid contributors within our society.

At the start of grade seven, Josh participated in all Special Olympic sports for the St. Albert Special Olympic team. It is by far the most exciting pastime for Josh. In the summer he takes part in soccer, track, baseball, and swimming. Not only is he great at all of them, but he cannot wait for the games and practices. He loves to win, but can also quickly forget he has lost. Josh, like all Down's can be a poor sport, but only for a minute. He can be competitive, but only for a second. He can, however, love forever.

43

Never will he leave the field without hugging all who are present, winners and losers. He holds no grudges or jealousies for long, and is always smiling and ready to participate in all sports. He doesn't seem to get bored, as we, so-called "normal" people can. He respects and loves his volunteer coaches and would die for them.

These kids have a certain honesty and simplicity that separates them from all of us. Special Olympics, and these special kids, are the medicine for our family's soul. Our kids, Karen, and I, spend many rewarding days with the St. Albert Special Olympic program. Whether it's a dance, a party, a game or our offer as a family involvement in an annual baseball family picnic, or tournament, we, Josh's relatives, walk away from those activities with an invigorated spirit. It is a therapy that has enriched my children's lives, brought my family together, and given us a sense of purpose. It's a tonic of good and honesty within.

We have found a world of loving and caring that does not always exist in the "real" world of "normal" people. In fact, we have much to learn from these kids and how they approach life in general. All young people, at an early age, should spend time with Down's kids, as those who have grown and gone to school with Josh have. They would learn the virtues of sharing and caring and unconditional love, like the love that Josh has for his family and friends. That loyalty is something that is not present in our "normal" society, which at times does not share well, if at all. My family is the recipient and benefactor of this boy, and I thank God every day for having blessed us with him.

Special Olympics is an organization that fulfills the dreams and ambitions of all mentally and physically challenged kids of all ages. These organizations exist all over the country and are funded and run by voluntary donations in funds and in manpower, and to a lesser degree with help from federal and provincial governments. It is disgraceful the lack of attention they receive from the media, simply because they are not the stars who sell the required image in a world obsessed with beautiful people and commercialism.

They don't sell soap, clothes, cars, or other commercial products. St. Albert, where we reside, is the base for the St. Albert Special Olympics. The leader of St. Albert's Special Olympics is a most gracious lady, who exceeds all expectations of a volunteer. Wendy Stiver has single handedly transformed this project of love from a small "track meet" to a major event with over 300 Olympians participating, in a multitude of sports. She has tirelessly worked for these kids for over twenty years. Her unselfish and unpretentious attitude is a reflection of her sincere desire to reach deep within the very soul of each of these kids and make their lives as rewarding as possible. She organizes every sport event, for every season, for all the kids. She is responsible for the coaches, the venues, the transportation and the social activities on a daily basis, twelve months of the year.

 She asks nothing for herself and gives all of herself for the kids with whom she works. They, in turn, respect, and adore her, thinking of her as a second mother. Her love for them, and theirs for, her radiates with every hug she gives and receives. She is "Special Olympics" in St. Albert. Her reward is nothing more than the love they feel for her. Her leadership is an inspiration to us all. My family, in part due to my wife Karen, has been sold on Wendy and the program. My wife volunteers all of us for duties, and for all of my kids (as I have already said), it's a blessing. All of our lives have been touched by the time we have spent with these kids.

Moreover, it has made us a better family, working for these remarkable kids. It takes courage to live the lives they do, yet they

45

smile always, love everlastingly, hate never, and completely enjoy every thing they take part in. I used to think of myself as a hero whenever I accomplished something on a sports field. When I place myself in their shoes for just a while, I know I cannot walk that mile in their shoes. The kids with special disabilities, with insurmountable mountains to climb, are the real heroes of our society. They should be the poster children for all of us, as they exemplify everything that is fair, good, sharing, loving and caring in this world of ours.

So many people have made and continue to make a contribution to Josh's mental and physical development. Literally all with whom they come in contact contribute to the mental and physical capabilities of Josh and children like him, and an increase of their learning curve. Josh is spontaneous and yet reflective. He remembers everything, especially those things and people about which he cares dearly. Josh enjoys sleepovers at his sisters and will engage his sisters at every opportunity to get invited. He enjoys going over to Jodie's house in part because Jodie is especially perceptive with Josh, but also because another one of my sons-in-law, Gage, Jodie's husband, is available to him. Gage is responsive to Josh's needs and treats him as an adult. He, too, has a special affinity and deep affection for Josh which radiate from him.

Josh loves Chris and Gage as they have literally taken over some of my responsibilities regarding his development. He loves them because he knows they are genuine, caring, fun, and most of all honest and yet disciplined with him. Josh can sense who really loves him and who are pretenders. These children have an uncanny ability to analyze eyes, grasp at your soul and know the truth about those with whom they deal on a daily basis. They love Wendy, their St. Albert Coordinator of Special Olympics because they know absolutely that she has unwavering love for them and would rather be with them than anyone else in the world. Josh also has a real closeness to Karen, my wife and no wonder: she is his physical, mental, and emotional rock. He knows that when all else fails, his mother will never fail. Strangely enough all our daughters also realize that their mother is the "music" that rocks our family and keeps it in tune with a balanced dose of perspective on daily life. She will be there with unconditional love for the rest of his and their lives. Karen's drive and desire to look at the worst but see the best, at the poorest and see the richest, in life in general, and Josh in particular, has made the difference in his life. As I keep stating, it takes many people from all walks of life to bring out the best that a special needs child can offer. Josh offers a lot, perhaps much more so than most people, but he has also been given much.

There would be no discord, if all people of the world were a little more like Josh and less like who they presently are. Our older daughter, Shawna, has had six miscarriages. Many discussions have taken place about that and we have always assumed that Josh has not followed all the conversations nor understood them. During one of our regular Sunday family supper (a weekly happening for us, thanks in part to Josh's insistence when it first started), Josh invented a game where each of us would answer one question about each other, our work, sports or any other issue he perceives. On this particular evening the first question was for Shawna and related to babies. He asked if Shawna would like to adopt a baby someday. Until then, we had not noticed how much Josh listens, and that he is aware of much more than we care to think. It was real awakening for us all. From that day forth, every Sunday, Josh has a game during supper, where he asks each and every one of us a question of the day. The questions are printed from the computer and I must say relevant to our weekly problems and happenings. We look forward with anticipation to his questions and are excited as to what our questions might contain. It's never dull, as any questions on any issues can ensue.

Spontaneous situations initiated by Josh at given times in our lives have been always led to warm hearted fun stories. One day, I was coming home from school at about 4:00 PM. Pulling into my crescent, I heard and eventually noticed a police car followed by a fire truck in turn followed by an ambulance and a police cruiser tail gating me. They wanted to pass, but were unable to because of the bottleneck as one enters Heritage Lake, my crescent. They were obviously in an urgent state and signaling me to move over. I immediately turned left into my crescent, confident that they would continue straight down the main ring road. To my surprise they turned into my street right behind me. I felt very uncomfortable, but I had just three houses to go before I reached my house at the end of the cull-de-sac. I hoped once I entered my driveway they would continue down the crescent and I would finally get out of the way. They pulled to a screeching halt in my driveway, right behind me, circling my car, with the police officer quickly swinging my car door open and pulling me out of the car. The fire department was ready to get to work, subject to my answers. I asked them if it had to do with my speeding and I looked rather confused at the excitement. They asked me if I owned the house and did I know if anyone was inside. They also stated that someone in distress had called 911 from inside my house. They stated the person who made the call seemed to say that he was in some difficulty and was home alone. They could not completely understand the caller but needed to get inside quickly.

When we got to the front door I realized that I had forgotten my key, therefore we had to go around the side of the house. Luckily the side door was open and I didn't have to use the key, which I could not produce. I, along with the police officer, the paramedics and all the fire department entered the house. I walked onto the back landing, made my way into the hallway and eventually into the family room, calling out at the same time; no one answered. Collectively, we inspected the kitchen area and the nook. No one was there and no one answered. I decided to go to the basement, and once again officers followed. I reached the bottom step and looked to the right hoping not to see something drastic. I could see my daughter Paula on the couch.

I gingerly walked towards her hoping, holding my breath, praying, that she was fine. I reached her and called to her; no response. I shrugged her, and at first, no response, but soon after that, she awoke and slowly tried to decipher what the commotion was. She was alarmed and panicked as all the officers surrounded her. I quickly asked her if she knew where Josh was. She replied that he was upstairs somewhere. With the police officer, the fire fighters and emergency response unit right behind us, Paula and I ran up the stairs to the second floor and the master bedroom. The door to the master bedroom was closed. The police officer stressed that he should go in first, "just in case". I wasn't sure what he meant but "just in case"; I relinquished. He turned the knob and swung the door ajar. When the door finally opened there was Josh, lying on the bed relaxed and calm, watching a TV program. The officer suddenly yelled, "Josh. It's Josh from Father Lacombe. The Down's boy I told you about, who pulled the fire alarm and cleared the school, but refused to go out himself. It was -40 C that day."

Everyone broke into laughter, and the episode turned into a cheerful reunion for the police officer. The officer gave Josh a stern lecture and when questioned, Josh said that he happened to press the rotary button used by us in case of emergency. The officer also stated that they would let us go with out a citation but should it happen again they would have to charge us the mandatory $500.00 on false alarm. All ended well and we were lucky this time. In fact, I have stated before that at times Josh, without a firm realization of consequences, has placed himself and us in severe danger to say the least.

One cold, lazy, early Saturday morning, we were all asleep. Josh got up and as he has done many times previously, went downstairs and made what we thought was breakfast for himself. A while later he came upstairs, walked into Jodie's room, and woke her up to announce the patio was on fire. Jodie brushed him aside and told him to go back to bed. He insisted, and Jodie, on a hunch, decided to get up and investigate. When Jodie made her way down the two flights of stairs and went into the kitchen family area, she noticed that the shades had been pulled down and saw a silhouette of what looked like flames.

She decided to open the closed curtains realizing that we had never shut them before; therefore, it must have been Josh. He always did that, when watching his favorite movie, to stop the sun from coming in and reflecting against the television set. In a panic, without thinking, she stumbled to the upstairs area and into my room, screaming "fire". I awakened from a dead sleep, and in a state of confusion, tried to slow Jodie down so that some logical answer would come from her lips. She continued to yell, "Fire downstairs". I, in my shorts and bare footed, sprinted down the stairs and made my way towards the family room I did not have to go too far to see the flames visible on the outside patio deck. By this point, the flames had engulfed the area just outside of the family room. I remembered thinking that unless I did something, the house would most certainly catch fire and we would lose everything. I tried to go out the patio door but could not because of the flames. I ran to the side of the house, barefoot and in my shorts, without any plan of action.

As I arrived at the back, the flames were well on their way to a major fire. I started to throw snow and sand from the back yard on the flames. The girls and Josh, who were by this time in total panic, were looking for water and the fire extinguisher, all to no avail; as it was winter, all the hoses were purposefully disabled for the winter. I told Paula, who was outside with me, to call 911 and the fire department. While she was scrambling to do that, I continued helplessly trying to stomp out the fire by throwing snow on it, but it hadn't snowed for weeks and it was nearly impossible to find enough snow to smother the flames. I had to do something, realizing that the fire department had just been called and sounds of sirens were not heard…

I suddenly got this crazy notion that if I could go onto the patio and throw the couch, which appeared to be on fire, over onto the grass, I might be able to save the house. Without hesitation or further thought, I stormed onto patio lifted the flaming two seat couch over my head and like a projectile, heaved the couch through the air, with all the strength I could muster. As the ball of flame flew across the back yard, I realized that, in haste, I had thrown it right over in the direction of my daughter Paula. She, with some skill, ducked and avoided getting hit by the fire bomb. Finally, the fire department arrived and quickly smothered both the fireball and the wooden patio floor, which at this point was well on the way to destruction. We had averted a crisis. No one knew what happened and Josh insisted that he had not done it. By coincidence the same crew of firemen and the same police officer that had visited us earlier during the false alarm by Josh at school, and the 911 call previously at our house, were at the scene. While they did not know us very well, they all called Josh by name and said hello to him. They knew him well. Too well.

They investigated the situation and, while Josh still claimed he was innocent, the police officer continued to ask Josh if he started the couch on fire. He claimed that he hadn't, until the police officer asked him if he had lit anything on fire. Josh calmly replied that indeed he had lit the newspaper on fire, which he had left on the couch. Josh and the kids like him are not always able to make logical connections. He didn't see that because he started the paper on fire, he was the cause of the couch catching on fire. This theory was proven when the officer asked Josh again, if he had started the couch on fire, and once again Josh said that he had not.

He had only started the paper on fire, and he was comfortable with the answer, as according to him it verified his innocence. He was not lying but simply could not and did not make a connection between the two events. Another terrible situation had been averted, but in the back of my mind I began to realize that Josh should be watched much more closely while he developed skills necessary to recognizing the danger of specific situations. Many more episodes were to occur which would remind us all of the fragile nature of his mind. We dodged a bullet that day, but would there be others? And in fact, there was, not to long afterwards!

One morning a few months later, an early warm Alberta summer morning, with birds chirping and geese flapping out on the small cozy pond to the back of our house, once again the house was quiet; we were all enjoying our last fragmented early morning final dreams.

Shawna, my oldest daughter, who was up ready for work and making her final preparations before going down, heard crackling on the main floor. She went down to investigate and saw the reflection of flames and smoke billowing towards the front door, making its way towards the upper house, having engulfed the kitchen and family room area, which were situated at the back of the house. In a panic, she yelled "Fire, fire!" All of us, who at this point had previous recollection of the same screams, quickly arose from sleep and without hesitation ran for the main floor, ready to face perhaps something worse but hoping for the best in process. Shawna arrived first with Jodie right behind her, I was slightly in back of her and the others followed. Nothing was visible, as the smoke had engulfed the whole kitchen, family room, and nook area, a rather large area at the back of the main floor.

The kitchen table and chairs were on fire. Shawna and I quickly scrambled for the water at best we could and Jodie desperately searched for the fire extinguisher which, after the previous fire, had been placed in the kitchen area, just in case. It was the fire extinguisher that helped snuff the fire and saved the house for the second time. Had we not had the extinguisher not much could have been done to stop the fire from spreading to the rest of the house. Much smoke damage was evident, two chairs where charred, the table was no longer usable, the curtains were ashes, the floor was scorched, but the flames were smothered and the situation under control. Fearful of what the fire department would say or do, we neglected to even call them as the incident took place. We had little time to contemplate in the panic. They were, however, called later, as the insurance company demanded a report from them.

Once again the same fire personnel showed up. This time they sat Josh down and literally scared him straight by threatening a jail term. We did the same as we had done the previous time he'd started a fire. A mock arrest was arranged for maximum affect on Josh. A fine was almost a reality but dropped at the last moment.

From that day on Josh seemed to learn what could or would happen should he repeat such action. While we remained vigilant, Josh learned from the experience and to this day has never involved himself in any more fire activity.

Doug DuCharm is a wonderful young individual, who exemplifies the best of young people, through his willingness to help people like Josh. As he had done so many times in elementary school with Josh and other special need students, he asked if he could become Josh's doubles partner in tournament play against other schools and "normal" kids. The very first time it happened in elementary, I was excited and overwhelmed with the care that Doug showed Josh. Just to offer to play with him risked Doug's reputation and left him open to harassment from other students.

The day of the game all of our family made an appearance to lend support to Josh and Doug. At the start of the game, Josh, who normally is keen, but not nervous, seemed to be just that. He could sense the importance of the event to himself, Doug, and Mr. Sorochan, the badminton coach who had suggested participating in the tournament to Josh and Doug, and to us. The speed of the two players in comparison to Josh was evident, but Doug, who was a top athlete, would not let it bother either of them. Josh made some mistakes, but you could see as he became more involved he not only felt more comfortable, but also more encouraged by the events taking place. The second game went much better. As a matter of fact, Doug and Josh won the second game after losing the first.

The third game was close. Oh so close! I was tense and reacting to every play, mentally playing the game with Josh at every move. Doug dug in and kept encouraging Josh and working with him in his positioning, movement of his feet, and wrist action…Josh was sweating profusely, as he often does, but it was much more evident in this game. All the spectators realized that this was unique and special. They asked if in fact Josh was Down's, as his performance suggested otherwise. The fans, players on both sides, and all the coaches were glued to Josh's court and attentively observing and absorbing every move. Josh and Doug were playing with one heart, united as one it seemed, and Josh responded to his mentor with all he had to give.

They lost, but on the last play of the game, to give the other team a win by two points, which is the requirement of victory. Despite their loss, a standing ovation awaited Josh and Doug. I was ecstatic with Josh's play, but even more thankful to Mr. Sorochan for believing in Josh, and to Doug for his unselfish desire to give of himself so that Josh could experience an exciting moment in a normal game, by and with, and against, so called "normal" kids. Integration was at this point alive and well on the basis of all that had transpired. The two boys against whom they had just finished playing also sensed how special the event was, as they came across and congratulated Josh and Doug for their courageous effort. Karen and the girls were in tears, not only for the effort that Josh put in, but for the care that Doug showed and his willingness to be a true friend. Josh hugged Doug and Doug reciprocated. I hugged Josh and in turn Doug, while the whole family hugged Doug for the courage and unselfishness he showed in the handling of the situation. To Josh, the implications of that day were not as visible and clear as they were to the rest of us and the audience, but his happy, sparkling face reflected his gratitude and appreciation towards his true friend, Doug.

JOSH'S HUMOR

Because of constant concern for Josh's mental development, we enrolled him in an enrichment class for the arts at the University of Alberta, specifically in a painting class. When we got there on the first day, I noticed that all of the children were of Asian descent. When I asked why, they told me that the class was set up for the benefits of the sibling of the University Professors. I was also told that these were the most gifted kids. I became a little apprehensive at the thought that Josh would be socializing with intelligent kids and not able to keep up, but I owed it to Josh to at least have him take part. The class went well. The students quickly perceived Josh's status and were generous and helpful with him at every turn. They shared with him, instructed him and channeled him in his attempt to paint a flower. It was a unique and rewarding experience for Josh and after the class ended, all of the children came to Josh, introduced themselves, and encouraged him to come again. The teacher stated that they had never shown that kind comradeship and that having Josh in the class would be a rewarding experience for the other children. When we got home, my wife, Karen, asked Josh if he had a good time. He replied, "yes". When asked if there were any other Down's syndrome children in the class, Josh calmly replied, "Mom, they were all Down's. Just like me". Karen turned to me and asked, "Were there any other Downs?" I said, "They were all Asian, but Josh thinks they were Downs." We both broke into laughter.

Can't Hold Me Down   Joe Petrone

CHAPTER
6

Grade Nine Grad

That Josh would even make it to the grade nine graduation, was both satisfying and unexpected. With all the dooms-day forecasting by every doctor and social worker at Josh's birth, it seemed strange but a pleasant surprise that Josh would attend a graduation, and even more difficult to imagine that it would be his. Many years had gone by with many wonderful events (and some not so wonderful) that to actually, finally, be able to witness his graduation would be a thrill for the whole family. Josh was as proud as any student at the prospect of his graduation and all of us looking forward to it. He and his sisters shopped for some comfortable slacks and a shirt that would give him some normalcy and belonging.

They found some rather mod teenager dress shoes which he would not wear, preferring to wear what all the other kids were thinking of wearing, runners. His preoccupation, like all other boys, rested with the question of a date for the dance. It was easy; his Down's friend, a very sharp, beautiful, close friend of the family and a girl that Josh had befriended at the Special Olympics events. She might be the girl. In fact, he wanted to ask her himself without help from us. She accepted and the date was planned to its minute detail. Megan, his sister, was also graduating and her reactions, excitement, wishes and anxieties were all the same as his. The day finally came. It began with the graduation portion of the night, a presentation at the school where all of the kids would be called up and introduced as graduates.

Megan, a real leader and a friend of many members of the student council for the school, was chosen as the Master of Ceremonies for the evening's proceedings, and she would be instrumental in making sure that Josh would avoid any mine fields that night. Her friends, who all knew Josh and had gone to school with him during the past eleven years, (including preschool) would be on hand and they, too, would be a blessing for Josh, as they were prepared to treat him as a friend. Our whole family bought tickets and many of our friends did as well. Everyone wanted to be part of the progress that Josh had made to date. All of these parents who at times had doubted whether Josh was deserving of graduation, were now convinced of the power of integration and assimilation. As a parent, it was rewarding that Josh's classmates, administrators, teacher and teacher assistants would be so accepting and fraternal with Josh.

Their collective support was obvious the moment Josh's name was announced and the call was made, by his sister Megan, for Josh to come up to receive his grade nine diploma. A standing ovation awaited Josh as he strutted up to the stage; he knew he had accomplished something special. He showed poise and confidence and carried himself with a certain comportment. All of his sisters and Karen sobbed at the emotional ovation he had received. Even I had to compose myself to avoid crying. Josh also received a special award for fair play, and kindness to all, and had to go up again. And again he was greeted with a tumultuous response from those assembled.

Afterwards, parents and teachers came to us, to personally congratulate us for the work that all of our family had done with Josh towards his upbringing. I was quick to point out that without Karen's and my daughters' dedication and love nothing could have come to fruition. Little did they know how much their sons and daughters had also been instrumental in his growth and development during the past eleven years, a fact we were quick to point out to any and all whom we engaged that night. The second half of the night was the dance. I, as usual, was concerned at the prospect of Josh at a dance without supervision, especially with his sister attempting to do her thing, and possibly ignoring him the whole night. I conceived a night where he and Jan would be overwhelmed and neglected, if not scorned.

My fears were totally ill founded, as Megan made certain that everyone of her friends danced with Josh and Jan. He had a great time, and at times his hambone and showmanship surfaced on the dance floor, as he literally led the rest of the students in a dance that is called the "Josh-step" to this day. When I picked him up at 11:00 that night, he was beaming, for he knew that he was accepted and liked, not for how he looked on the outside, but for his heart and soul inside. He was proud and so was I. I started to ask him questions and he quietly answered some, but not all. A rainbow of colours shone from his eyes and a smile of pure happiness was on his face. He knew that he fit in and all was well. He could see that I was happy and that was swell. When we got home, he looked into his mother's tearful, but radiant eyes and he knew that she, too, was proud. The love and pride that his sisters felt that night, was never in doubt. After all, he was a sixth sense for them. He is truly their Prozac blanket, with a special awareness of their preoccupations, their daily frustrations, and their pensive, tense moods, as they walk through life's daily stresses.

JOSH'S HUMOR

One day after Josh and I got home from his daily work with the hockey academy, we were sitting at our kitchen table ready to have lunch. Josh was busy operating his calculator, trying to come up with a specific sum of money. Shortly after, he said to me, "Dad, I have spoken with Paula and she tells me that if you die I will get a lot of money. Can you tell me how quick this will happen so that I can get it? I really need it so I can buy Jan a present." I replied that only God knows when our time is up; therefore, we must pray to him for things we need. He replied, "I will pray extra this week".

Can't Hold Me Down

Joe Petrone

CHAPTER
7

The High School Years
Grade 10

We never imagined that Josh would ever get to grade ten, and therefore high school and Josh's eventually graduating seemed so far fetched and so far away that it caught us by surprise. Josh's entering into a new phase of his development made us both apprehensive. Our trepidation was increased as we considered the prospect of his entering a new, larger school with many students whom he did not know. We worried about the size of the kids, the different mine fields that he would have to navigate as he matured, wanting to be "grown up" and become a productive member of society.

As a high school teacher, I had a vision of things to come and the frightening prospects for Josh, a boy without hate, malice, worldly knowledge or understanding of the unknown. His trusting personality, his desire to be liked and accepted could be detrimental to him should he be in contact with that small group of individuals who would try to do harm for no specific reason, other than to satisfy their crazed concept of fun.   We were also apprehensive about the teaching staff who dealt specifically with his independent study program, as they were new to him and new to us. We were skeptical but anxious to move on. The summer months before Josh began high school were a refuge for us all. The prospect of his upcoming challenges was totally forgotten as Josh enjoyed all of his favorite activities in the vicinity with people who loved him and cared for his well-being. Josh was involved with Special Olympic Soccer, basketball and baseball practices. Sprinkled throughout the summer were many soccer and baseball tournaments, scattered all over the province.

The final and most awaited tournament came up in late August in St. Paul, Alberta, where all the provincial baseball teams meet and fight for the Alberta supremacy. Josh loved, lived and dreamed baseball. He was, I must admit, one of the top power hitters and players in the province. He has an uncanny ability to hit home runs, and he hits them a mile. Because of all of his hits in the St. Paul tournament, he is called "the king of St. Paul." He invites many friends and relatives to travel to the games, and any one else who cares to be invited.

Josh's attachment to the Blue Jays is something fierce. He is one of their most enduring fans. He watches every one of their games on TV. He knows every player, every stat and every trade within the ball club and throughout the whole league. He duplicates all of their moves, including their pre-swinging tirades, spitting, scratching, grabbing, bat handling, chewing and any other irritating contortion and tension-reducing action that all players engage in during the game.

He is also immersed in track and field during the summer months, and there too, a provincial meet takes place. He is entered in many events, including 100 meter sprint, long jump, relays and most of all, the shot put, which is his strength. An innocent observer would not be aware that he is Down's by the way he throws the shot put. He is superb in it, and with hard work, in which he's prepared to engage, and some top coaching, he should be able to reach the national team level, and be a member of Canada's Special Olympics team, if one exists...

Then, all too soon, the official orientation letter arrived from St. Albert High School, and it seemed that we had gone through this before. We were to report to a designated classroom on the first day of school for a meeting with the Individualized Study Department, so that the teachers, students and their parents could get together and be taken through an orientation regarding the next three years. There we were, early, so that we would get a front seat and be part of all discussions. The class was starting to fill and everyone was filing in. We scanned everyone who came, to see if we could recognize anyone. As it turned out, many or all of the special needs students Josh had worked with and had gone to school with from preschool to grade nine were there, as were their parents. All of the teachers, of course, were new and soon we would meet with them. The class was called to order and we parents attentively sat, hoping to hear and feel comfortable as we did during Josh's junior high and elementary years.

The teachers were dignified and well versed. The program seemed to be of high quality. The teachers were professional throughout, but we did not see in them the enthusiasm, warmth, or love and affection for the kids that we had seen in junior high and elementary. We were in high school, where teachers are more objective, if not slightly distant towards most, if not all, the kids.

The room was cold, the atmosphere too business-like; however, even more of a concern was the idea that these kids would not have an assistant assigned to each of them but one for four of them, who would rotate with each student as the need required. Josh would have to go to many classes without the help of his assistant but only the care and attention of the teacher in each of the classes, who would be too preoccupied by overloaded classes and a full curriculum.

As a teacher faced with this very situation, I knew how difficult it would be for the teachers to cope with as many as five special needs students and a whole array of difficult, so-called "regular" kids. In this atmosphere it is difficult for any teacher to really produce a top-level class atmosphere, regardless of his or her expertise in the field. However, the funds were not there for specialized attention and that was the reality of the day. In many cases during the first year, these kids would be participating in an integrated program without the individualized help when required. Because of Josh's and all other special-needs kids' latent development in relation to other kids who were now to be fellow students, total integration would not to be productive. Compounding this was the fact that, in most of the courses, into which Josh was placed, the difference in the learning ability of his classmates in relation to Josh, was too drastic.

You could say that Josh, and all the other special-needs kids, had reached the point of diminishing returns as to learning. Participation in most of the classes would be relegated to physical appearance at best, with very little understanding of most of the lessons that were given. Realizing this, we decided to modify Josh's timetable with those courses which he would not only enjoy, but with which he could connect and be an integral part of. Josh was given physical education, drama, religion, computers and food study, all courses in which Josh not only excelled in, but enjoyed and could participate in while in an integrated environment. Josh spent his first year doubling up in physical education, drama, and computers. With the help of many teachers who were not assigned to him, Josh also participated in intramural floor hockey, basketball, badminton, drama, the year play and music.

The students of St. Albert High School exceeded our expectations, for they spent time with Josh, worked with him, paid attention to him, and cared for his needs the best they could. When Josh was asked to play football by the head coach, with a coaching staff prepared to work with him, I decided against it, knowing full well the problems he would face in the heat of the game. Having played the game of football, I was concerned with the dangers that football would pose for him. He did, however, participate in the school's track team, in the shot put, and in the official school badminton team, just as he had in elementary and junior high.

During the first year at the school, Josh worked hard and intermingled not only with other students within his special program, but also established a reputation with many of the normal kids as a good athlete and a nice person. Josh's involvement with physical education and his athletic prowess whenever any game was played in those classes allowed him to reach many of the so-called athletic kids of the school, who made him part of every game they involved themselves in. He was asked to participate in noon hour floor hockey, which was a competitive sport played by all, and a large part of the inter-noon hour recreational atmosphere in the school.

Many games were played and spectators watched as teams competed for the coveted intramural championship. One of the top teams, made up of top athletes within the school, drafted Josh to play on their team. When I was told by the physical education teacher that this had happened, I thanked him and said that I would like to personally thank the boys for their gesture, but that Josh could not possibly play to the requirements of the high caliber, fast moving game that I knew would be played. He replied that what the students had seen from Josh during the physical education classes convinced them that he could not only be a part of the roster, but was fully expected to take a regular shift and play an integral part in the success of the team. The fact that his peers had invited him to participate was an exciting prospect for Karen and me, but Megan, who played on another team (the games were co-educational) did not look forward to having to play against Josh's team.

The day that Josh played Megan's team, Karen, myself, and all our kids, went to the school to watch them play. The gym was full of students supporting one team or the other. The additional story to unfold was the presence of Josh, who had by now made an impact on everyone who went to the school and had heard stories about his antics at the school and during these games. Josh was a real showman. His warm-ups, his skill level, and his flamboyance contributed to Josh's acceptance by the other athletes, the students, and the teachers watching the game. As I looked around and observed, I realized that Josh was the center of this game's universe and that he was truly a show by himself. A halo-like aura seemed to surround him.

He not only scored goals on this particular day, but interacted with the other players just like any athlete, and showed grace, desire and love for the game and his teammates. His teammates took it all in stride and made him feel like an equal. The fans cheered and clapped at any gesture, emotional maneuver or skill that Josh exhibited that day. After scoring a goal, he took off his shirt and raced around the gym, with "high fives" for any and all present, including his sister, who was on the losing side. Megan's friends cheered for Josh and showed sincere spirit for him. We, as parents, never envisioned such a day or such events could ever have happened to Josh. The honesty, courage and friendship that the boys had shown for Josh that day remains a pivotal testimonial to the power of eliminating hate and ignorance, and to the truth that integration can work, if all kids, educators and parents work with, live with, share relationships with others of different faiths, ethnic and racial backgrounds, and those with physical and mental shortcomings. Schools, work places, and society in general can be much more caring and sharing, helping to make this a loving planet that all of us can enjoy.

Can't Hold Me Down   Joe Petrone

JOSH'S HUMOR

As we often do during supper, we were discussing and digesting events to come, when I mentioned that when the proprietor of a chain of top end Italian restaurants in Edmonton was in possession of Edmonton Oilers Hockey season tickets, and that he occasionally gave them to handicapped organizations for kids like Josh. Josh is a real hockey nut, and a true lover of the Edmonton Oilers. He loves to go to a live game when the opportunity arises. That night Carmelo, the owner, of the Sorrentino's chain, called, asking for me, and Josh answered the phone. When Carmelo asked if I was home, Josh replied, "Are you the man with the free Oilers tickets? If you are, and have some for me, I will call my dad to the phone".

Can't Hold Me Down   Joe Petrone

CHAPTER
8

The High School Years
Grade 11

Josh's grade 11 year progressed at a fast pace with few hitches. He had set into the routine of daily high school life. He had befriended all those in his individualized program and many of the other students. The teachers and aides were responsive to all that Josh attempted and more than willing to give him a hand. He in turn, was always prepared to share with and care for everyone he met. He was asked to report on sports events for the school newspaper and given a post within the student union as an official special-event assistant, nametag included. While to us, a special event assistant might seem a meager role, to Josh it was a confirmation of their trust and affection for him.

He showed up at every meeting and work detail and made it his duty never to let anyone down. The principal of the school, a close friend of ours, with whom both Karen and I had gone to school, gave Josh a special seat in his office, which Josh utilized on every occasion, usually every day and sometimes more than once a day, to inform of anything happening around the school, with the usual dosage of rather interesting suggestions on all issues.

By this time Josh had established that his relationship with Jan, a gracious, loving young girl, would with her parents' permission, actually transcend from a friendship to a much more loving connection between the two. Josh melted with her appearance and doodad after her every wish. They shared everything, like any normal, loving, high school couple. They went to dances, parties and family get-togethers as one. They frequently went to the movies driven by one or another set of parents. I was frightened by the prospect, but the wishes of Josh and Jan, along with everyone else in both families won the day and the ritual of Tuesday movies came to pass. Josh fastidiously took her coat, helped her to the car and closed the car door for her. He walked her to the door and asked me to park slightly away from the house so that his good night kiss with her would not be noticed or disturbed by me.

Josh quickly found out, however, that relationships with Down's were no different from other kids, as Jan did always what she wanted to do (or else!) on every occasion. They only went to movies she liked and approved of, and she insisted on being picked up exactly on time, regardless. When Josh arrived, usually he had to wait. Josh lovingly complained to me one night, asking why Jan was late. I replied, "Welcome to the world of living; now you are like all the other men in this world". He didn't understand but laughed at my answer. He is prepared to sit and wait for Jan, as his love for her is mature and sound to him.

In the spring of his grade 11 year, Josh continued to play and be a part of the school track team and a guest player on the badminton team. While the teammates and his coach were willing to accept, and have someone play with, Josh in a regular match, we all decided that Josh would only play at the exhibition level, where the situation could be less traumatic and more educational for Josh. In track and field, however, Josh did take his place on the shot put squad and exceeded all expectations.

He was the only mentally challenged person to ever be part of his normal high school athletics team. Regardless of the outcome, neither the rest of the athletes' coaches nor and of our family and friends wished any more of Josh. He had accomplished more that we could ever imagine. As he stood with the other athletes to receive his participation medal and picture taking, we noticed that he felt proud that we were there, and his shining face was aglow with happiness. His teammates were also proud, for they lovingly embraced him as one of them. That truly was the greatest reward for Josh, to be accepted and loved by his peers. As Karen came close to me, we hugged and I softly said, "To be loved by their peers is what all humans strive for and glow at receiving and dread never being embraced by it, in their frail young lives." On this day, physical appearance was not an issue but a blessing, for Josh was accepted for his worth inside of his heart and mind, in this daily walk of life. Josh has never been intimidated nor labeled himself Down's. We and society have labeled him so. God has simply placed Josh's trust in us and it's our mandatory duty to guide him through the many crossroads of life, for God's gates are entered not by race, color, and/ or physical appearances, but by our daily deeds of love and sharing with our fellow humans.

JOSH'S HUMOR

Our neighbour and friend goes away during the winter months. These winter months require someone who will clear the walks as it snows often. He asked me if I knew someone who would or could do the job while they were away. After a major search to no avail, we decided that Josh could do it. For one thing, it would teach him discipline, and most of all he would get fitter and strengthen his heart. I asked Josh and he said yes, but asked how much he would make. I told him that it would be great for him and he would receive $100.00 per month for the five months. Josh also has numerous other sports events he has signed up for which he must attend. During this particular winter it snowed almost daily, and as Josh was not available I became the official snow shoveler. In late March with a few more days to go according to the contract, Josh happened to be out with me shoveling snow. My friend, the owner of the house, had returned for *a week on important business. At this time, he decided to pay Josh the total sum owed for the year. Josh was quite excited at the thought of five $100 bills in his hand, he thanked him and as my friend left for the airport, we continued to shovel. I looked up and saw that Josh was walking toward our house. I called out to him reminding him that we had not finished our job. Josh replied, "Now that he has paid in full, you handicap, there is no reason to do it anymore. We have the money in our pocket, why get cold for nothing?"*

Can't Hold Me Down   Joe Petrone

CHAPTER
9

The High School Years.
Grade 12

Josh's grade twelve year suddenly came upon us. It was much anticipated, but with guarded optimism. This was to be Josh's last year at school and we started with a pensive look into the plans that he might make after graduation. Josh has always demanded a certain amount of freedom and individualism. He has dreamed of a day when he could make his own decisions and perhaps live his own life, rent his own apartment and yes, even marry some day. To him, this seems a possibility, but to us, sadly, it seems an impossible dream.

We were inquisitive as to what type of job Josh could and would hold after graduation. Josh's strength on a job would be his congenial, trusting, smiling, happy, attitude…Josh would struggle if he had to devote himself to a normal, daily work plan, as his concentration span would not allow him to be of service for a long time. Nor would Josh work well in an atmosphere of deadlines, antagonistic everyday stress, or in a competitive field.

Josh does not really understand finances or all that money can accomplish in our daily lives nor does he understand the devastation of being without it. At all of the part-time jobs he has held, Josh has never been paid, but he is undeterred by that prospect, nor does money fit with his vision of work. Josh works well and loves situations where a fun and congenial attitude are part of the work experience. He also brings a certain amount of pride to his work and to things that he does in general.

When his first day of Grade 12 finally arrived we were invited to the high school to meet the teachers, parents and students. While he knew all the students from his individualized program and had many friends within the "normal" program of study in the high school setting, a slight curve suddenly was thrown. His program was the same as usual, but most, if not all of his teachers had changed. The program of study in the high school setting had created some difficulties for Josh because of the variety and the demands of courses that he had to take in order to graduate. More academic courses, in "normal" classes with "normal" kids. Moreover, the teacher assistant that was assigned to him had other responsibilities and could not be in each of his classes at all times. This meant that for the first time, Josh would be in a full "normal" high school environment, without, in our opinion, the guidance and security of a trusted person to take him aside and channel his thoughts. Special needs can be vulnerable to outside suggestions if supervision is neglected. The courses that Josh really liked and excelled at, such as physical education, food science and fashion design, were not available to him, as he had already taken his share of options. Furthermore, Josh was expected to fulfill the requirements for specific courses such as math, English, and other academics without any of the individualized help that he had been blessed with in his previous years in school. A few frantic calls were made to the school by Karen and myself but ultimately everything worked out for the best, as Josh rose past our level of "un expectation" and quickly adjusted to his new demands with vigor and enthusiasm.

As in past grades, Josh's outgoing personality was infectious and soon he met and socialized with the same vigor as in his past years. Josh was even granted a small part in the year play, as he took drama. Josh also had a class in fashion design and loved it, mostly due to the number of girl registrants. All of them took a real liking to him and loved to chat and show sincere friendship for Josh. Josh is known, as most Down's are, for their love of hugging everyone they come in contact and socialize with. It is their way of showing friendship and affection. The girls loved it, but I was a little concerned, constantly wondering what an 18-year-old boy might do, faced with the possibilities. However, never once did we have a complaint about an inappropriate act by Josh in any of the social situations throughout his school years. As a parent, however, the response to all of the social elements leading to sexuality is to worry. Josh, and kids like Josh, are naïve and do not understand the stress that sexuality can place on a young boy, with or without Down's. Throughout his school years we continued to hope that Josh would learn to respect the privacy of others and never place himself in an inappropriate behavioral sexual dilemma. Karen and I worried, and continue to do so, about any episode that might some day lead to a complaint of a sexual nature. Should it ever happen, I know Josh and kids like him are not malicious, for they don't really understand all the implications of biological sexual needs.

Josh continued to participate in intramural floor hockey, on the same team as in the past years, and did well as usual. He once again tried out for, and became part of, the school track in shot put. Once again, he did spectacularly in this event. He threw better than in previous years and performed so well that he did not finish last in his event, which was a monumental feat. The majority of the athletes who threw in his event, upon realizing what they had witnessed, showed admiration for Josh and his physical achievement of the day. When Josh was born, our vision of his future was a daily process. Our preoccupation was short term and our expectations from what we were instructed to dream for Josh, were a daily event at best. Never did we imagine or comprehend to what extent Josh could soar, with a little help from everyone with whom he would eventually come in contact. Karen and I were surprised at his grade 9 graduation and the top marks that he received. It was a stretch to even contemplate that Josh could and would graduate with a high school diploma.

Even more breathtaking was the thought of the actual graduation itself, if and when it came. Well, folks, in fact it came: Josh would graduate with honors in his individualized grade 12 program, a very respectable feat for a boy, that the medical establishment of old had dismissed as not possible. How many thousands of children have been sacrificed and at what cost? Few people recognize the capabilities of Down's children, especially with the love of family and friends. The unwavering faith of Karen, our children, and the concerned, sympathetic, devout educators in the human spirit, proves the importance of a small investment of care and trust.

At the graduation ceremony, Josh would be an integral part. He was to receive two awards, an honors award for an average over 80 in his class, and a service award for his congeniality and his love for school, the students and life in general. At this point, Megan, who had been in the same grades with Josh throughout their school years and, was graduating with a very strong average, seemed to be forgotten in our enthusiasm for Josh; however, we had learned long ago, at the start of Megan's voyage in the same grades with Josh, that she could handle it. Megan was a rock throughout the many years with Josh. It was Megan who witnessed and heard the daily stories, and at times Josh's actions embarrassed her, yet not once did we have a negative response from Megan towards Josh and his educational roller coaster. Megan showed maturity beyond her years in the handling of Josh. It was not expected, but certainly welcomed and appreciated by us.

I have felt anger and frustration at times, during Josh's travel through the educational portion of his life. It was I who had, and at times still do have doubts, about the potential that God granted Josh. It has been I who has been the fatherly worrier for Josh and conscious of his every action, both in public and at home... It has been I who has found the most difficulty with my lack of confidence in Josh's ability to progress.

It has been I who has tried to protect Josh from the outside world, wanting to spare him harm and ridicule at all cost. It was, and still is, my wife Karen, my kids and my sons-in-law, who have allowed Josh much more freedom and space to experiment, try new ideas and grow. It has been Shawna, Jodie, Paula and Megan who have given Josh the wings to fly, and the confidence and courage to do so. My kids have given Josh the will to go forward and taught him to dare to dream of new possibilities. It has been they who loosened the rope to allow Josh to go where my protective clutch would not have taken him, and it is because of them that Josh has surpassed all expectations.

Our collective family, including all of Josh's cousins, who have treated Josh as one of them, allowed him to demonstrate his worth. At every turn and every party, they have embraced and trusted him. Their patience, loyalty, friendship, and mentoring have allowed Josh to experience a normalcy that only they as peers could provide, yet also gave him the compassion and protection he needed. During Josh's visits at our family cottage, where all of the family spent many weekends, the nurturing and care for Josh was most evident. All of his cousins respected his space and created an atmosphere of growth for Josh which was gratifying for Karen and me. Karen, my kids, and all of our immediate relatives, including all of Josh's cousins, have always allowed Josh to feel, smell, visualize and explore the path for himself, giving him the confidence and ability to meet and defeat the next challenge on his winding road of life.

It is natural for a father to react in a protective manner, as I have on many occasions. As a teacher, I didn't want Josh to become a prey of all the hurts that humanity could wreak on a young, innocent, person. I was steadfast in my pursuit of a Shangri-La for Josh, hoping to spare him any possible harm. The truth of the matter is that parents of all children must resist the temptation to smother and stymie. In spite of our sincerity a sprinkling of tough love is necessary to ensure individualism and discipline.

The Merchant's hockey team, one of the strongest in the Junior B hockey system in Alberta, is one of the many stimulating aspects of Josh's growth. He has been asked by the team's coach, my son-in-law, to help out as best he can with servicing of equipment and other related items. His number one responsibility is to supply water to the players during the games. Chris, the coach, told him that his handling of, and supplying of, the water for the players during the game was crucial to the team and more wins would be possible because of his help. Josh took his duty very seriously, absolutely convinced that his contribution for the team was important. It allowed Josh to socialize in a game where all members and participants were normal.

This is huge for the Josh's social development. Chris also had him taking stats as well as assuming other hockey duties during the games and then reporting the outcome to him in between periods. This was not important to Chris but was precious for Josh. He was so excited by the team that he followed, the team on the Internet, and still does to this day, and usually knows every stat on the team and players. Josh will never forget a game. His attachment and devotion to the team and the players will not allow him to. The players have taken a liking to Josh and not only care for him but treat him as an equal. The socialization and interaction that Josh experiences is crucial to his self-esteem. Every fan knows Josh, and he has become the symbol of unity for the team.

Josh always purchased the nightly 50/50 and has won on many occasions. The players and the fans realize that Josh is keen on the tickets and all hope for him to win. Josh is equipped with a personality that everyone enjoys and wants to be around. His humor and wit, which borders on sarcasm at times, is refreshing, funny and warm.

On March 15, 2004, Josh finally became a man, at least according to him, when he turned eighteen. Every time he asked for a drink the reply from all of us was always that he would be able to drink once he reached the legal drinking age. He was looking forward to his birthday, since Josh, like all other kids who dream of adulthood, knew that then he could drive, drink, smoke and go to the bar. The girls always told him that at the age of 18 he would be entitled to do these activities without permission, as a consenting adult. On his 18th birthday we rented a pub in St. Albert where Paula, one of his sisters, worked. We invited 150 of his teachers, administrators, caregivers, friends and relatives. They were all excited to come. Most came with presents (lucky for them, since Josh waited for them at the door and asked each of them if they had brought a present).

A good day was had by all and Josh drank a little and got somewhat light headed. I had not told our family that I did not agree with Josh's drinking, nor that I wanted to discourage it. All ended well however, with everyone having had a great time. Many made speeches, including the principal of his graduating high school, who spoke of how wonderful his experiences with Josh had been, especially those many days when Josh went into his office to ask him if he could assist him in running of the school and determine his opinion regarding the problems that had to be rectified.

The principal went on to tell Josh that now that he was 18 he could do adult things, like drinking, without interference from anyone and without worrying about the police, so long as he did it responsibly. The next day, to school he went, and during the lunch break, Josh and his girlfriend Jan went to the cafeteria for lunch, sat down, opened their bags and took out their lunch. Josh also took out two Coors-Light, my son-in-law's favorite beer, opened both and passed one to Jan. They were both calmly drinking when one of the teachers realized what was going on.

For a while, she could not stop laughing, but she approached Josh and asked him where he got the beer. He stated that he got it from home, that he had more and asked would she want one. As they were talking, another boy came by and Josh asked him if he wanted a beer. The teacher quickly put a stop to it and asked all concerned to report to the office immediately. She did not want to report Josh, but felt that at least a talk from the principal was in order. Josh replied that the principal knew about it, in fact, it was he who said at my party, that I was an adult and could do what I wanted." When the principal asked Josh why he had brought beer to school, Josh stated that he was 18 now and could do all he wanted without interference from anyone. They all laughed, but a lecture was in order on why what he did was wrong. . Meanwhile, Josh became a folk hero to the students, as the story spread like wild fire. Everyone looked for Josh to congratulate him, as the other students thought that Josh had pulled off something they all would love to do someday, but never would.

JOSH'S CARING

Domenic Mobilio, a former Edmonton Driller Player and top scorer, was living in Vancouver when he suddenly died of a massive heart attack on the way home from a soccer game he had just played. It was a shocking event, which sent all those who ever played with or against him to Vancouver, to pay their respects to his family. I was made aware of the distressing news by another one of our players at the time, Carmen D'Onofrio, who also resides in Vancouver. I had been Dominic's general manager and signed him to play for the Edmonton franchise.

More difficult for me was the fact that, during the last year of our team's operation, we traded Dominic to Philadelphia, granting him his wish to make more money and receive a guaranteed contract which we were in no position to offer. The trade was by far one of my lowest moments in my soccer playing, coaching and/or managing life. With his death, the memories of rancor and doubt once again resurfaced. Even more captivating was the fact that Josh, who was never told of his death directly, but as usual, was very observant of any conversation or action that went on, suddenly walked up to me and in a soft tone made me aware that he had a picture of Dominic, which he had asked for and been given by Dominic personally, at one of our family-player get-togethers. I looked at the picture and indeed it was of Dominic at his best on the Coliseum turf, ready to score goals. It was not autographed, but it didn't matter. Josh went on to say, with mist in his eyes, that he had written on the back of the player card, "One of my favorite players and he promised me he would score two goals".

In fact after some checking, we found Dominic indeed scored two goals for Josh the next game. Josh has never forgotten that gesture or any of the positive relationships he had with all of the Drillers who spoke with or visited with him. He was adamant that we send the player card to Dominic's family. I told Josh that Dominic would want him to keep it, but that I would relay the story to

Dominic's parents and relatives when I sent a condolence card to them. None of us, including myself, had any idea that he even possessed the card, nor that he had the intuition to react to and understand the gravity of such an event.

Can't Hold Me Down   Joe Petrone

Can't Hold Me Down   Joe Petrone

CHAPTER
10

The High School Years
Grade 12 Graduation

The day that we wished and hoped for, but never really contemplated would be a reality, was suddenly, by the grace of God, thrust upon us: Josh's grade twelve graduation. After celebrating a teen's 18th birthday, this is the next most important event in the lives of young people and their families and friends all over North America. It was official. The letter from the school suggested that Josh had earned his place as a member of the 2004 graduating class. Upon reviewing the letter, I noticed that in fact, Josh had successfully completed the Independent Living Skills Program, actually received his certificate through hard work and determination.

The graduation was to be on May 22nd, the same day that Megan would also be graduating. Her mother and sisters worked with Megan towards her goal for that evening, as there was never any doubt of her potential or her level of success. Without too much notice, they had made all the arrangements and she was well on her way to the most important event in the lives of all young people and I must admit, parents.

I, as a teacher, had to witness many graduation ceremonies in the course of my duties. I had never been enthusiastic about my grade 12 graduation, which I had not attended, preferring to play a soccer game instead, and for that matter, I never attended my convocation at university. My parents, who pushed me to excel and get the education that they could not achieve, were neither aware of nor culturally involved with the notion of graduation as we practice in this country. They never asked me about my grade 12 or my University graduation. My diplomas in both cases were sent to me by mail. Moreover, coming from a background where wine was served at every meal and major occasion, since I was a toddler, it wasn't so important for me and my family to await with anticipation my 18th birthday, so that I could over-drink and make an idiot of myself, either pretending to or not remembering any of all that had taken place. It seems that this tradition is very important to North American teens, who have been told over and over since youth that drinking is bad. In many states in the U.S., young persons are asked to fight for, and often literally give their lives for their country at 18 years of age, but are not allowed to drink until their 21st birthday.

We were brought up in a culture where drinking as a family and at the supper table or at special events could be responsibly done and enjoyed. I have always allowed my children to have a glass of wine at supper, as my dad did with me, and I have found that my kids were not fixated with the notion of drinking or being 18 to drink, and, therefore awaiting that day with great anticipation. Drinking does not consume their lives. Josh was somewhat different. As the girls made it a point to illustrate to him the virtue of waiting till 18 before he could drink, Josh had been waiting with excitement for his 18th birthday, with rather amusing consequences as a previous story has so amply described.

Now, as Josh's graduation day drew nearer, the girls were determined that this would be a day that Josh and all of us would fondly remember. Many days prior to the awaited event, the girls collectively decided to make certain that Josh, at his graduation, would have all that the other graduates hoped for and more. They took him to the finest places in Edmonton hunting for leather shoes made in Italy, escorted him to numerous clothing stores in search of the best shirts and pants, and decided on a fine tuxedo which both fit and made him look the part. They also made certain that Josh made all the required arrangements in the form of transportation, flowers, and after-shave. A manicure was also arranged, as was a trip to his special hair stylist.

As the day drew near, we also had to worry about the needs of Megan; she too was graduating with honors and had an illustrious career in her high school years. We knew that Megan would understand our need to fuss over Josh with less reflection on her needs.

The day of the graduation came, with the church ceremony slated for 7:00 PM that evening. My wife and kids planned to arrive at church early, so that seats could be saved for all the relatives and friends who had wanted to take in the festivities with Josh. A whole row of church pews was reserved and as some of our people scheduled to sit in them were late, a small problem of saving the seats became an issue with other parents who were at the church but had no seat. It did not matter; my family was ready to face any issue for Josh's night. The church ceremonies went very well and Josh took part in all of the activities planned for graduates. Most, if not all, of the people in church that night, knew and had followed Josh throughout his school career, and were delighted at his special day. Everyone was cooperating in the delivery of the events to embrace this night for Josh.

The next day, we were off to the Jubilee Auditorium for the introduction of the Graduates and the receiving of their diplomas. We all sat there in our seats waiting with anticipation and pride, as the Petrone names were called up, Megan was first and she walked up calmly and relaxed. She smiled and looked radiant and she, too, knew that the next name to be called would receive huge approval. A little resentment on her part must have crossed her mind but she did not look annoyed or angered at our embracing Josh's day in the sun. She understood so well that her success was appreciated and loved by all of us.

Megan had created her own following at school, and her success was evident by the calm reverence that her teachers and friends demonstrated toward her at every turn. The graduation banquet and dance was to follow that night. Megan and all her friends had arranged a limousine to pick them up and take them to the events of the evening, while we brought a super new Lexus to drive Josh and Jan to the proceedings. At five o'clock Karen and I, along with our remaining daughter, picked Josh up from the hair stylist and got him, perfectly dressed, to the car and off to pick up his girl Jan.

There was so much to worry about that we all forgot the corsage for Jan, and so we had to detour and enter the flower shop and literally help the employee make one, as she had run out of them.

We were a little late, but the wait was worth it. Josh and Jan looked smashing together. A perfect couple. Josh was so consumed by his attention to all the details that he had to follow with Jan. Karen and the girls had trained him in all that he had to do when sitting, walking, holding a lady's hand and dancing with her. Everything was rehearsed and planned out by them, for Josh. We arrived at the banquet late and everyone was worried as to what might have happened. Our table was in the center of the hall and we had to walk past many sitting guests who were just starting to eat. Josh walked so proudly, and Jan seemed to follow all his gestures and overtures. When we got to the table, the questions as to where we had been were answered and we all sat down for the meal. Josh walked over to Jan and softly pulled out her chair for her to sit, and then calmly went to his seat for the presentation. Everyone, it seemed, was staring at Josh and Jan with approval and love, as they had by now managed to make a difference in the lives of many of the people in the audience, including all of us, his teachers, administrators and all of the students.

When he switched his seat, refusing to sit by me, I knew he was concerned that I would be overprotective as to what he could eat, what he could not drink, or with whom he should or should not dance. I made a promise that on this occasion I would defer to Josh's wishes and avoid smothering him at every turn on this very special night for him. It was his wish, and I was prepared to stay back and allow him the freedom, to finally explore, open up his heart, relax a bit and be himself. During the presentation, his picture and his name were shown and mentioned at the podium. A cheer went up as his name came up in speeches made by different dignitaries. The night was glorious and exciting. He and Jan looked fantastic together. The best couple there.

Josh and Jan danced all night with each other and a sprinkling of many teachers and other students who wanted to dance with them. Josh and Jan never left the dance floor and Josh's card was filled for every dances. This was to be a culmination of a success story that had started in preschool. As Karen and I finally sat there in the midst of all our great kids and friends, with time, for the first time it seemed, to sit back a bit, away from the glitter of lights, cameras flashing and music playing, we both felt a moment when we could let our guard down and contemplate what Josh had achieved. What might have been, had he not been born to our family, or gone to the school or received the guidance from so many wonderful people who had taken Josh as a little boy and guided him to adulthood? All of those people who dared to dream and take the challenge, so that someday Josh would be where his night had taken us all.

All of Josh's caring teachers were heroes that night, as they all had been working for his educational development. They all deserved a hand shake and a medal for their efforts with Josh, not for personal gains but out of compassion for a young boy to whom they were committed, with the love and affection that all teachers hope to give their students. On this night, all of the people there, including many of the parents of those children at our preschool meetings whose kids had shared all of Josh's educational years with him, had contributed to Josh's success. These people, with my wife, my kids, my sons-in-law, Chris and Gage, had shaped Josh into the man he had become.

The unconditional love, true friendship and service they have shown in the rearing of Josh to the man he is cannot be repaid. As I stated before, it takes a village to raise a "normal" child, it takes a very large city to raise a Down's child. On this particular night the hall was the village and the city, for it took all of the people there and more to give Josh the help to prosper, thrive and achieve and become what he is today. Josh has many more hurdles to jump and many more of what seem insurmountable mountains to climb, but what he has now is the ability to face them with the confidence to jump the hurdles and climb the mountains.

Karen, his sisters, Chris, Gage, and all of our relatives and friends gave him the tools and the courage to jump and to climb, while Josh has the heart and soul to get to the top, having learned from his mother that the sun will always shine on top of the mountain and God will await and hold his hand every step of the way. Josh can soar now, for he can fly with the wings of confidence that have been granted to him by Karen and the kids. He will have set backs, but he knows that his mother and family will be there for him.

I have learned so much from Josh about my own strengths and shortcomings. As a father and as a person I too, will no longer walk in front of Josh, but slightly behind him every step of the way. I know I can let go of that rope and watch him soar and fly away. Not completely away, but just enough to give him space and freedom to feel the independence that he cherishes. Yet I will remain ready to help, and to give him the confidence to do it alone. My wife knew, the night he was born, that this day would come. I could see it in her eyes that night, a strange reflection of God's will into the future. In retrospect, I also knew that night that while I had my doubts, she remained determined that all would work out for the best, as it has. She knew; and her prayers have been answered. She knows through her spiritual connection to her God that nothing happens by chance and that all is planned by God. Everyone is called, and some can see it clearly. For others, it takes longer, but all will hear the call, see the sign, follow the light and help their fellow man, before their time has come.

Can't Hold Me Down   Joe Petrone

JOSH'S HUMOR

One day I picked up Josh after one of his instruction sessions on sex education, given by Special Olympics, for the purpose of making certain that all the athletes are educated on the proper attitude towards sex, as well as its implications and consequences. After the session, I asked Josh, as I so many times do, what had happened in the class and what, if anything, had he learned. He replied, "It was a about a lady having sex with her doctor and then a baby came out and the pictures looked disgusting and some weird sex was going on." Josh really is not quite certain to this day what real sex is all about and he was taken aback at how babies come into this world. His concept of sex is taking off your shirt and kissing your girl. He has not grasped the full implications of sexual activity. We hope that this course will help him develop some understanding of, and a healthy outlook towards sex, love relationships, family and the outcome of babies.

Can't Hold Me Down   Joe Petrone

CHAPTER
11

Josh Today

Now that Josh has graduated from high school and is well on his way to manhood, he indeed is making a contribution to society. He has been hired by the office of Special Olympics as a "go-to" person in the office. He washes dishes, cleans the floors, shreds paper, stamps letters, mails them, and opens mail. He has a small office desk, which Carmen, "the boss" as he refers to her, has opened up for him so that he can rest his body and relax on occasions when he is not busy, and feel like a part of the staff.

His time there (three times a week) is a blessing, as he loves to go and cannot wait for those mornings. Like any other person, he anticipates the events and attempts to dress accordingly. He fusses over his hair, makes a solid attempt at shaving, and is more diligent with the type of cologne he uses, (which at times is way too much for any occasion and enough to kill anyone in his vicinity).

One morning while he was washing his hair, I suggested to him that he and I should be using a different kind of shampoo that his mother Karen had purchased for Josh and myself. I said that it was "less costly". He simply stated, "Dad you are already married and can use cheap shampoo, but I have to marry Jan and she wants me to have shining hair not cheap looking like yours".

Carmen and the rest of the staff work hard to treat him as they would any other worker. He likes that and appreciates it. He loves Carmen and respects her suggestions and recommendations.

All that has happened to Josh seems to be the work of a superior power, as Carmen, many years back, worked for me and I can easily say that she was organized and disciplined in her work. She is a superb role model for Josh, with plenty of guidance for him, but also with a small measure of tough love with him which is sometimes required, as it is with normal kids. Josh has continued to be an integral part of Special Olympics and still participates in all their yearly sports and activities with a sprinkling of dances as a social outlet for the kids. Wendy is still there with her leadership and love for these kids. More than ever, Josh follows the Blue Jays at every opportunity. His unconditional love for the Oilers has given him much needed excitement as they traveled to the Stanley Cup finals in the 2006 season. His exuberance throughout the play-offs was slightly doused by the final game and the final loss by the Oilers. They came so close and went so far, but to Josh this was a small glitch to another season of fantastic loving hockey to watch.

Paula, our third daughter got married to Kent our third son-in law on September 16, 2006. He, too, is a friend, role model and a favorite of Josh, as the other two son-in laws have been and continue to be. Josh has already invaded their house with visitation rights and stay-overs.

Josh continued to impress those he had met for the first time through all of the weekly wedding requirements and Paula's marriage ceremonies, by acting and being that normal person that everyone was used to. He danced all night, was a favorite of all the guests and a little flamboyant as only Josh can be. Paula was a truly radiant bride and together with Kent looked and acted like royalty at every turn. My father-in law was a little taken aback by the lack of an official Catholic celebration but enjoyed the proceedings as he, a 90 year old, and Josh, Down's, were the only two people standing for literally all the dances.

Now that I have officially retired from teaching and am in transition, while in the process of writing this book, I give Josh rides to all places on all occasions, making me as he exclaims "his taxi driver". On days when he does not work with Special Olympics, Josh will spend time doing much the same in the office of PetroFin Manufacturing, a company that has been set up by my nephew for the manufacturing of pre-insulated copper and other tubing for commercial, industrial and residential applications. With supervision and respect, Josh can work any time in any situation. He has grasped the tools required of any person during his upbringing, school experiences and social integration. He has learned from family, friends, associates, and the public in general, what he needs to play a meaningful role in society, demonstrating his own worth to himself and honouring the expectations of others.

Josh's preoccupation at the moment rests with his passion to marry his sweetheart, Jan. He talks to us continually of it, meets with Jan and goes over any and all preparations he has imprinted in his brain from personal experiences at his sisters, weddings. He has spoken at length with Jan's mom on this topic and they seem to be receptive of the idea. But she, too, isn't convinced of the outcome. He has had many discussions with my daughters and sons-in-law on this issue and further has sat down with Karen on a specific course of action to bring marriage to Jan into fruition. I have been the only person left out of the loop, as he understands that I could be more of an obstacle to his evolving ideas on marriage to Jan.

I have already explained my thoughts on the issue of marriage as not too practical an idea. I believe that a short ceremony can be had. Special friends of Josh and Jan, who have lovingly participated in their upbringing, from immediate families to teachers, teacher aides, close friends and all other caregivers, can be part of a special day reserved for Josh and Jan; they can live together in a group setting or with us in our family setting, allowing them the freedom and self reliance they aspire to and the comfort that all is fine, while a vigilant eye is kept open for them.

Regardless, their vision and understanding on the issues of physical sex is at best drastically limited and not about to get better soon. They both perhaps have some biological drives and wishes but not aware of how, where and when the possibilities exist. Another concern is that while Jan can have babies through sexual activity, we have not researched whether Josh has the potential of impregnating Jan biologically. We have had people suggest that Down Syndrome males cannot in fact impregnate, while others say that it is possible. We need to do extensive research with a doctor and other Down specialists, as to the reality of intercourse and impregnation on the part of male Downs. It is very important from the standpoint that for two Down's children to have a baby is hopefully not possible nor advisable if possible. Meanwhile and undeterred, they have already formulated a long list of invitees and computerized invitations. They have chosen the church, the priest to administer the wedding ceremonies in a Catholic setting, how many Lexus will be required for the bridal party, the food required and where it will come from.   Jan's mom is caringly somewhat in favor of this, as are my daughters. Karen, my wife, is not too sure, while I don't see and cannot visualize a realistic un-fairytailed conclusion to a future official marriage. I have read where a few official marriages of Down couples have taken place, but I know that those couples were perhaps at the highest level of intelligence for these children, and while Josh and Jan are respectively at a high caliber of intelligence for Down Syndrome, it's a stretch to suggest marriage without serious reservations on our part.

To Josh and Jan it would be official as they would enjoy all aspects without neither knowledge nor care as to its legality, and they would without reservation believe that they were officially married and happy for the rest of their lives. I have at times suggested to Josh that once married, he and Jan would have to live together for a long time. He stated that they could be together for a couple of hours and then Jan would have to go back home and he would see her in a few days again. I asked why he would want to be separate from her, and he stated that he would want to go to his sisters for a sleepover and spend time with Chris, Gage and Kent our sons-in-law at hockey, ball hockey, and Oilers' games, as well as watching afternoon CFL and Blue Jay games along with other fun things they presently do with him. Jan also wants her space and has asked Josh to take her home or, if they are at her house, for Josh to go home.

The future for Josh certainly looks fantastic as he has ever-loving sisters and close relatives. With his infectious personality he has cultivated many friends from past and present shared experiences with normal and special kids like himself. He has great work ethics and is responsive to the feelings and shortcomings of others. He is tolerant of others and their faults, which he does not see in them or in his actions.

The other day we took our clothes to the dry cleaners. We usually send Josh in unattended to simulate the experience as training for his future self-reliance. When he walked into the cleaners to have our clothes dry cleaned, the lady asked him if he was Down's Syndrome. He apparently told her "no". When he got back into the car to join Karen and me he said "that lady at the cleaners asked me if I was Down syndrome." "What did you say?" Karen asked him. He replied to her that he'd said he "wasn't". "Can you believe that lady?" he exclaimed. Karen and I smiled at each other at his remark. My wife from the start has allowed Josh to walk into self reliance- and confidence-building situations to allow him the ability to foster independence and the courage and skill to face the future with of the freedom he requires.

After all these many years I have come to realize that Josh is more than capable of standing on his own. My wife and kids realized it so much earlier than I. I continually need to reassure myself that all will go well for Josh, for he has mastered all that we had to teach, and what has been thrown at him, and more. Josh is now a man and wanting of manly things. I must allow him this and facilitate this for his future happiness and mine. The marriage that Josh and Jan want so badly seems more plausible now that my family and I have traveled--not in his shoes, but in proximity to them--in Josh's ever expanding life to date. He has no self-doubts. He is positive and confident in his physical and mental ability to face all future obstacles that life imposes. I'm working with all my being for the courage to see what he and my family have seen. I see more clearly now. I thank Josh. He has been an inspiration to me and all those he has met and is sure to touch in his exciting future to come.

JOSH'S HUMOR

One afternoon while Josh was spending some time at my daughter Jodie's house, Jodie decided that Josh had spent too much time in the house and it was time for him to go for a one mile run. Upon his return she would start a movie that they were planning to watch. Time went by, five minutes, ten, twenty minutes. At thirty minutes Jodie started to worry and decided to go and look for him. She walked around the neighborhood aimlessly with absolutely no success. Turning back she went down the walkway at the back of the houses, just in case. As she got within a few houses of her residence she heard talking in one of the well manicured yards, coming from the patios of a coworker of hers and an ex-teacher of Josh's. As she investigated further she heard Josh's voice. She walked into the yard and was quickly invited to come up to the patio and join them and Josh. Apparently Josh left the house, walked to the back ready to run, and realized that a party was in the works and a great excuse for him not to run. He was planning to return and eventually tell Jodie that he had run, as she thought he had done on other occasions. The neighbour stated that Josh had made a habit of joining them, and had done this on many other occasions when Jodie had asked him to run. On previous occasions he had always gone back and told Jodie that he had run. At times he can be a manipulator of events to his advantage.

Can't Hold Me Down

Joe Petrone

CHAPTER
12

Josh's Wish & Prayers For Shawna & Chris

After six miscarriages, and later many discussions on the possibility of adopting, my daughter Shawna and her husband Chris enthusiastically decided to adopt a child from the continent of Africa – with Josh's approval. They met with many agencies responsible for adoptions in Africa, and both agreed that their best opportunity would lie in the country of Ethiopia. Having met their financial requirements, they participated in a series of interviews and psychological testing through the agency, to make absolutely certain that their willingness to adopt was matched by their spiritual, ethical, and economic potential for parenthood.

Finally, after many months of exhausting work and jumping through hoops, they were classified as great potential parents. Parents with a love of children, and the ability to handle the journey they were about to embark on. Frustration grew as they waited for their call, nearly to the point of a loss of hope. Then, on the day that my second daughter Jodie gave birth to her miracle premature child, who they named Luke, Shawna and Chris received their celestial call – they were now officially the parents of two twin girls from Ethiopia. That very day at the hospital, while tending to Jodie, we were all told the much-awaited news. Josh was about to be an uncle, and his mother and I grandparents times three!

They received the girls' bios and pictures and were told that they would soon be given the official date for their travel to Ethiopia and the beginning of their parenthood. Another long wait ensued before they finally got another phone call. We were all overjoyed, and Shawna and Chris were suddenly engaged in preparations which involved the purchase of all that was required for not one baby, but two! Two cribs, two beds, and two each of thousands of other things which had to be obtained in a short time.

We were all involved, all baby stores were visited, and more was purchased than was actually required. All of the relatives from both sides of the marriage were helping out buying shoes, clothing, boots, hats, winter and summer clothing of all kinds. It was overwhelming, to say the least. Not knowing the exact size of the two girls made shopping for clothes difficult. From the pictures, they looked small for toddlers of 2 ½ years old.

Shawna and Chris now had to direct their attention to the trip, and who might be able to go with them. They would need a helping hand during such an overwhelming cultural, emotional, and physical trip to Ethiopia. Josh thought that he, as a future uncle to the girls, would be the best man for the job. We all smiled sympathetically, for it was Josh who on numerous occasions had asked his sister if adoption could be an option for her. Without a feeling of rebuke for Josh, we all agreed that my third daughter Paula would travel with them. She, unlike any other person on this earth, can adapt to any situation – as needed, she could be persistent, flexible, hardnosed, cunning, smooth, aggressive, loving, and forceful in pursuit of her goal. Her help would give Shawna and Chris precious time during the trip to focus on the task at hand with clear minds.

It was decided that, despite the cost, first class tickets were essential. It would ease the trauma of long travel, and let Shawna and Chris spend time bonding with the girls. At first these tickets were not available for all of the flights, but Paula worked at convincing the ticket takers at the airports of the need for first class. All responded, and the first class tickets were obtained for the entire trip there at no extra cost. On the way back the situation was the same, and again Paula came to the rescue and first class tickets were made available. The 29 hour trip seemed long on the way there, but it would prove much longer and more difficult on the way back.

After an uneventful arrival and takeoff in Frankfurt, they also made a stop in Amman, Jordan and then on to Addis Ababa, Ethiopia. After landing they took a cab to the orphanage, where they were greeted by a very polite and efficient lady who seemed to be the spokesperson for the orphanage, responsible for meeting the parents and introducing them to the much awaited twins. They were placed in a waiting room the size of most living rooms in Canada, and asked to wait. They were never allowed to go to the back of the orphanage, where approximately 100 orphans of all ages resided.

As they nervously waited to see their twin girls for the first time, the heat, jetlag, and nervous perspiration were evident on all three of their faces. Some time went by and suddenly a semi hidden door opened, and an absolute miracle took place as Paula filmed the extraordinary event. The toddlers were introduced to Shawna and Chris, and I will try to explain what unfolded, but I cannot do justice to the looks on the faces of the children and Shawna and Chris.

The girls were fantastically beautiful, more so than the pictures showed. They had dark, overpowering eyes, beautiful features, and were small in size. Pensive, confused, dazed, shaking like frightened puppies. Most of all, they were holding tightly to each other for instinctive reasons of self preservation and protection, which seemed so elusive at this point. Whatever Shawna and Chris said was repeated to the girls by an interpreter, but the girls stared, never flinched, and remained wide eyed, trembling, and frightful. They would be required to stay 11 days to bond with the girls, and the driver they had hired for the time kept speaking with the children as the official documents were signed.

They drove with the children to a nearby Spartan, low-key guest house where they would stay for the duration. The five of them were left to fend for themselves in a one-room accommodation rather small in size. From the first day, the children had to quickly adjust to a totally different culture, strange language, and three total strangers who were white, to boot. The children were cautious and respectful, but wary of all that was done or said. They never spoke a word themselves for the first three days.

Shawna, Chris and Paula used this opportunity of tight, frugal living conditions to start to foster a family relationship with the toddlers. They read to them, gave them baths, sang to them, hugged them, and taught them about the people at home in Canada who were awaiting their safe return. Through pictures, they taught them the names of all relatives, the house which would be their future home, the rooms, clothes and toys they would share in their new exciting life.

They spoke to the children in English at all times. The two children relied on their ability to speak to each other, and when they wanted to shut their new parents out, they carried on their own conversations in Amharic. Shawna, Paula and Chris new from day one that these were not simply their miracle children, but were absolutely smarter than any child their age back home. They soon recognized that with love and a fermenting of trust, so important to any relationship, the girls became more compliant, willing, and relaxed. They started calling them mom and dad, they would play hiding games and ball throwing games.

Finally, a spontaneous, phenomenal smile, diamond brilliant, radiated from their eyes. As Shawna, Chris and Paula showed their love for the girls, their reassurance, courage, self esteem and confidence sharpened, and the dreaded trembling, shaking, fearful, withdrawn, confused looks disappeared as suddenly as they had showed during the first encounter. After 11 exhausting and culturally trying days under the hot sun, with the lack of forgiving water, unfamiliar foods, boredom, and a longing for Canada, it became a test of survival. The one offsetting factor was the two pearls which Ethiopia had just released and entrusted them with, to hold, love and cherish forever.

The monotony continued, but the spirit endured. They read books to the girls, watched movies, and sang more songs – some of which they had already learned from the girls! They also again visited a more palatable Sheraton Hotel, with more western ambiance and a more calming atmosphere. The days moved on and became more bearable, the nights were cold in the desert air. Their driver was forever caring and sympathetic, truly reassuring not just for them, but for the girls.

The final day came almost shockingly quick, their bond with the girls becoming strong. The girls called them Mom and Dad, and Paula had become Auntie. They knew the name of every relative back in Canada, could recite the numbers from one to twenty, name animals, and even say "please", "thank you", and an assortment of other necessary English phrases. When the plane taxied and they were in the air, a certain sadness was visible in all of their faces. Ethiopia had been hospitable, caring, and most of all trusting. They had entrusted Shawna and Chris with their most cherished possession, their youth. Everyone was hopeful that they could give the girls what their natural father and their own country could not.

As the plane continued its journey further and further from the capital, the twins held tighter to Shawna and Chris. Perhaps this time, these new parents would not give them up, but hold tight to them and protect and cherish them forever. Their eyes, like at their first encounter with their new parents, were somber, and the same was true this time with Shawna and Chris. They found themselves holding and caring for the twins, and each other. When they cried "Auntie Paula", she too joined the scrum of love.

The stay over of 9 hours in Frankfurt was an important and much-needed time. The girls had to be showered and de-loused at least once. They didn't have lice, but it was a precaution. More protein had to be secured and downed by the twins and the adults as well. The girls clung to Shawna as never before, at times breaking out into a screaming cry, perhaps remember the past and not completely trusting the future.

Paula landed first class tickets with her personable skills. The comfort of first class allowed them all to relax, and allowed the girls to slightly over eat – all that the stewardesses brought, and more! It was a feast for the girls and an enjoyable time for the adults. On arrival in Calgary, a snag developed with tickets. Paula, for some reason, was not ticketed to be on the same 25 minute flight to Edmonton but to fly 1 hour later. The problem was averted as a man travelling to Edmonton, having overheard the conversation between Paula and the ticket taker, offered his seat. It was truly a fantastic gesture on his part. He knew what they had done and why, and showed his thanks to Shawna and Chris for their unselfish act of love for two beautiful kids.

Most of our relatives made the trip to the International Airport in Edmonton, in anticipation of the first encounter with two leading ladies. Karen and I stood there truly emotional and vividly shaken, with joy and anticipation for two miracles to come. The moment came, the doors swung open, and there they were. All tired, exhausted, but elated at finally touching down in familiar safe surroundings where they could finally let go. Their emotions boiled over, and the totality of what had taken place erupted into a loud cheer with a spattering of tears everywhere, including some by bystanders who were moved by the outpouring of a sense of love we all shared. Chris, a police officer with Edmonton city's finest, remained dignified and just hugged his kids.

The kids, who for 11 days would not leave their sight, were engaged, content, and accommodating with every kiss and hug had by all. The car trip hope was eventful as Mea again started to cry, for whatever her reasons. It was overwhelming, unstoppable, heart-crushing crying all the way home. She is more pensive, less guarded, less convinced, and more hesitant at what she sees, hears, and does. McKeely, more flexible and easy to please, is more smiling and is protective of Mea. Perhaps since birth she has taken the role of protector for Mea, on guard for her needs and wants. They have been home for just two weeks and already the crying has stopped. Their love and trust for their parents is very apparent, and vice versa.

The girls have bonded more securely, and developed a love for Murphy and Trooper, the house dogs. Chris, who is back at work now, calls every hour and misses his girls. They run to him as he returns. It's fantastic, in two weeks they have gone from strangers, to acquaintances, to friends, to a loving family. Their future looks bright, and blessed with what they truly wished from God.

While Shawna and Chris appreciate and can never repay Ethiopia and the girls' father for entrusting in them this gift of life, the grandparents (Karen and I, Rita and Jim Gallagher) want to thank, with all our hearts, the people of Ethiopia for their unselfish act of kindness for us. Mea and McKeely will appreciate their blessing, and the opportunity now given to them without strings attached by two loving and caring parents. I hope they grow strong, healthy and smart, and never forget their birthplace while accepting with love their adopted country and parents. I hope someday they both use their enriched future, with the gift of education given to them in their new country, to help their birth country out of their immense poverty, disease, lack of education, and everything else affecting Ethiopia today – things that our children take for granted, but which children in their own country will never experience or hope to obtain.

They are two precious and beautiful pearls, and priceless to Shawna, Chris, and us all. Much is expected from these two children, and much they will achieve. They are smart, witty, funny, caring, loving, and each has a splendid personality of their own. Their new parents, I know, will guarantee true and unconditional love. Their future is secure, God will see to that, and all else will rest with them.

Josh visits them at every opportunity. He helps to feed them, walk, and entertain them. He loves his new title of uncle and takes that responsibility to heart. The girls adore him. Perhaps they sense that he is, as they are, blessed and assured with the possibility of a productive and prosperous life ahead. Shawna and Chris have been and will continue to be superb role models for Josh, as they are and will be the Rock of Gibraltar for their two pearls from Ethiopia.

Shawna and Chris's prayers have been answered by God. Mea and McKeely's future awaits, full of hope and sunshine. Their dreams will come to fruition. Their love for each other and their new parents will forever grow. They will be missed back home, but they will be loved here, by us all.

Can't Hold Me Down   Joe Petrone

Can't Hold Me Down   Joe Petrone

CONCLUSION

The only person who could and should have written this book with full authority, writing in the first person, is Josh. Had he done so, definitely this book would have been much more anticipated and worthy of print... In fact, Josh has indirectly written this book, for it is not about his birth but rather the invaluable life experiences that he has shared with us so far. He has given us all a sense of purpose and stability.

Our family and close friends have come together because of Josh more than any other reason. Our daughters, two of whom are teachers (Shawna and Jodie) and one who has graduated as a nurse (Paula) and is presently working at the University of Alberta in the Cardiac Centre, are better equipped to deal with the complexities of today's world and educational and societal integration. His heart is huge, his smile is wide, his laughter is contagious, his soul Godly, innocent and pure. His love for his family and friends is a warm quilt, woven with labors of love, courage and strength. Josh is always happy and proud of his fortune, which the ignorant label a misfortune.

On many occasion he, has told us, "I am the luckiest person in the world, for I have the greatest family and life on earth. I love my life." We, who have shared a small part of daily life with Josh, are truly blessed, for it is we who have profited from his simple wisdom. Josh is a testament to early intervention, in a stimulative school setting, guided by innovative, caring, loving, understanding teachers, assistants and school administrators, who allowed him to grow and thrive as a contributing member of our society.

Anyone who meets Josh, even once, can never forget him. Josh is captivating. He is an angel of God. He is also a reminder of our obligation to our family and friends and our obligation to love and cherish every single day. Josh, like all of us, has had, and will have, his down days, his up days and his mad days; however, Josh does not dwell on past events, down events, or sad events. He does not complicate events or stress over them; he takes all with simplicity, honesty and a unique confidence that emanates from his hug-full body.

We should all strive to be more like Josh, for our lives and the lives of all people would become vacant of hate and distrust, which have caused numerous wars, killing millions of people and accomplishing absolutely nothing. In many ways, Josh is a reminder of our desire for a simpler past, when families were united in prayer and in deed; when a neighbour was a Godsend, not a curse; when a true friend was there always and doors were never locked; when family dinners were a daily occurrence, books were read, libraries were visited, people talked to one another and technology had not yet devoured our individualism. When pop was 5 cents, movies were 25 cents and Sunday was reserved for God and family. When Gordie Howe and Bobby Orr, Jackie Parker and Pele were true heroes to us all. We shall never see those days again; however our family and friends, teachers and administrators have been blessed with this reality every day, with Josh and his simple and unconditional love for us, which we can never repay. God got it just right, when he sent us his earthly light. His name is Josh.

Josh At 5 Months.

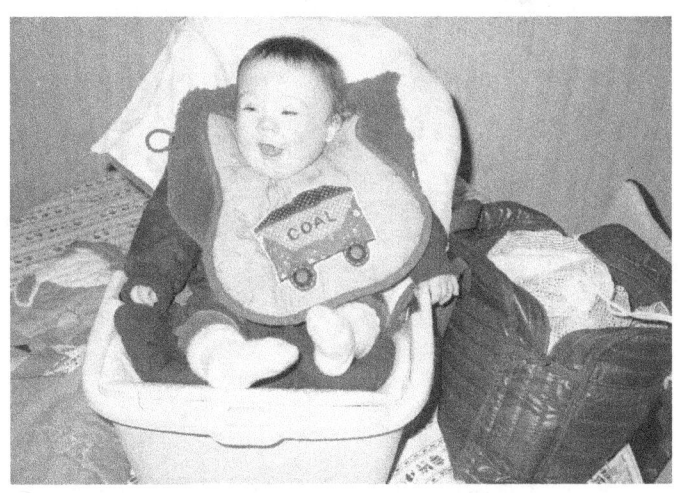

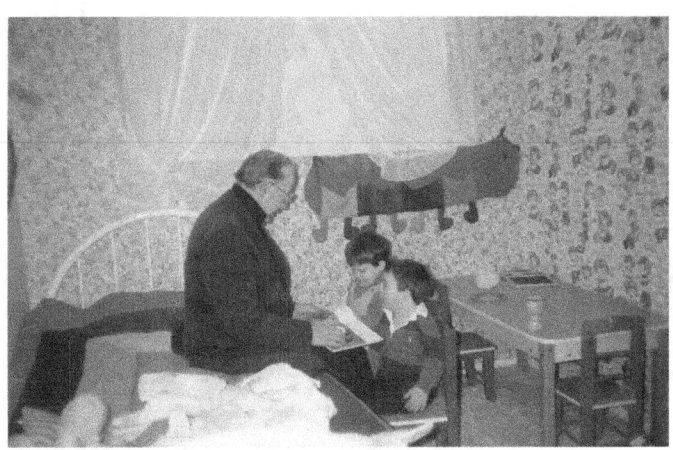

Grandpa McCoy reading to Josh & Megan

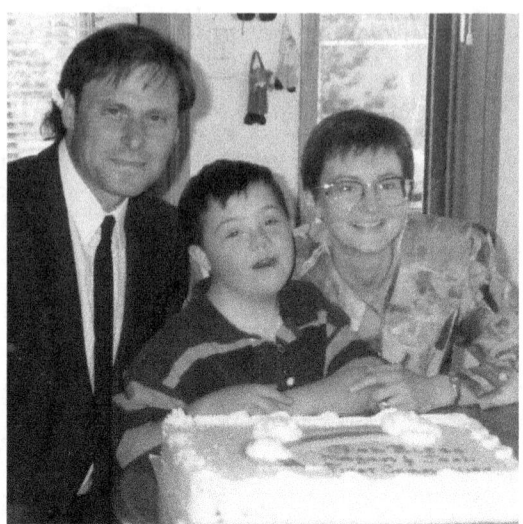

Uncle Tony, Josh & Auntie Carmen – First Communion

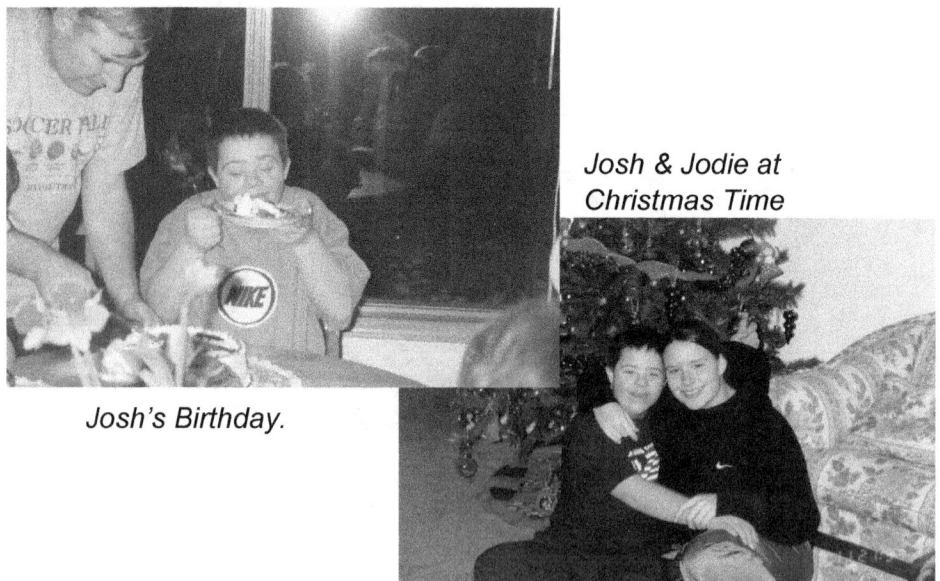

Josh's Birthday.

Josh & Jodie at Christmas Time

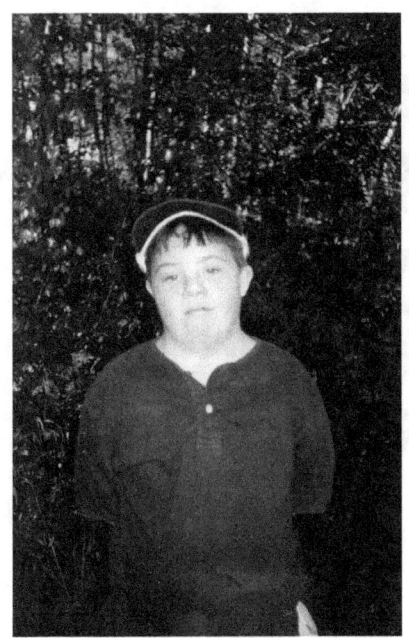

Josh at the Lake

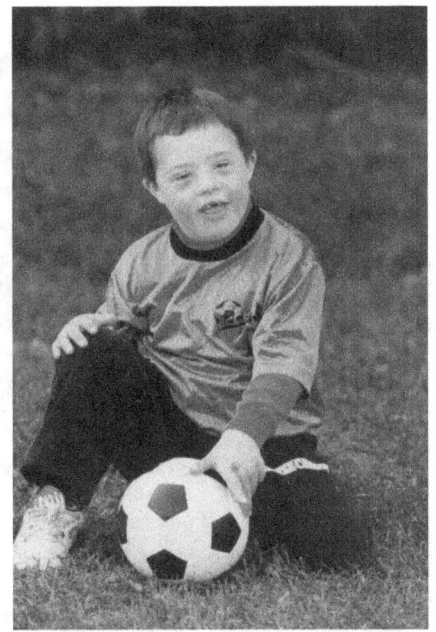

Josh Playing Soccer

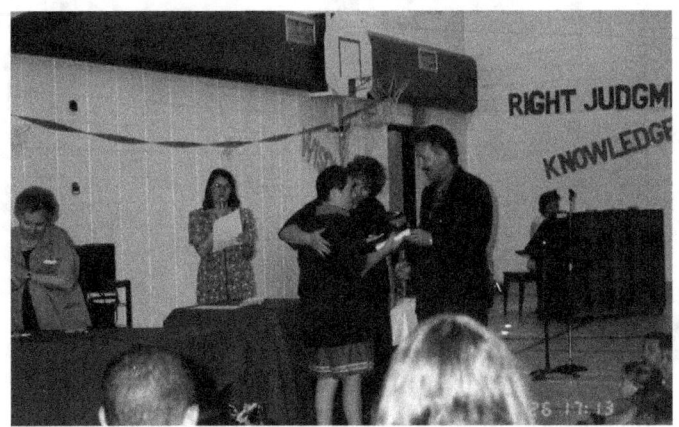

Josh Graduating – Grade 6

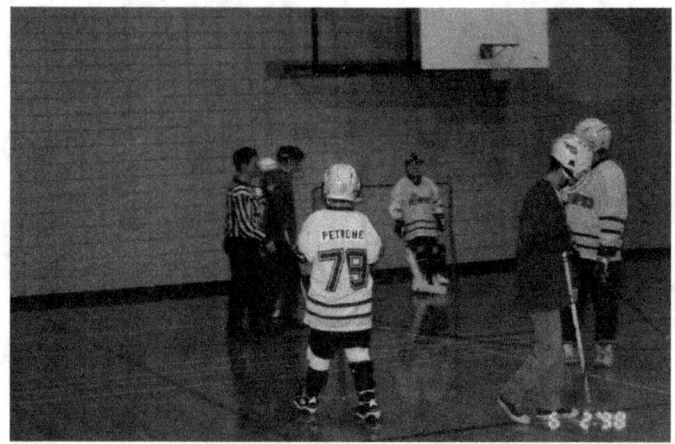

Josh Playing Floor Hockey

*Josh at Megan's
Soccer Game.*

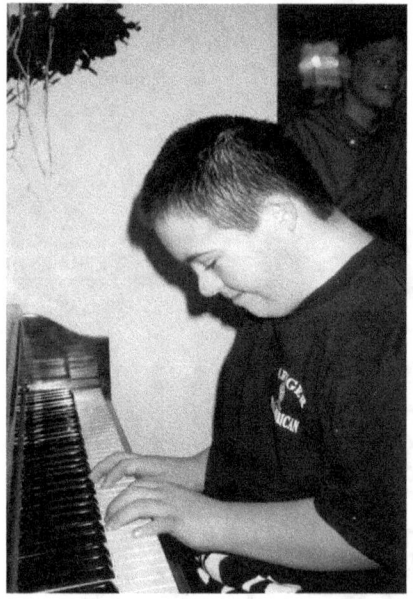

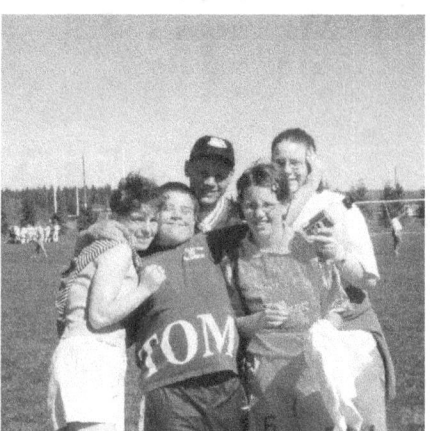

Josh Playing Piano

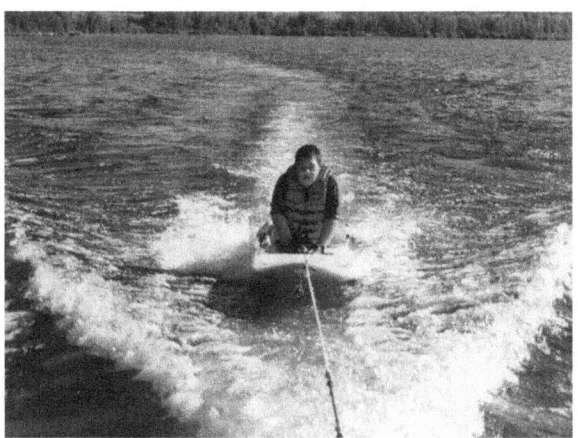

Josh at the Lake Tubing

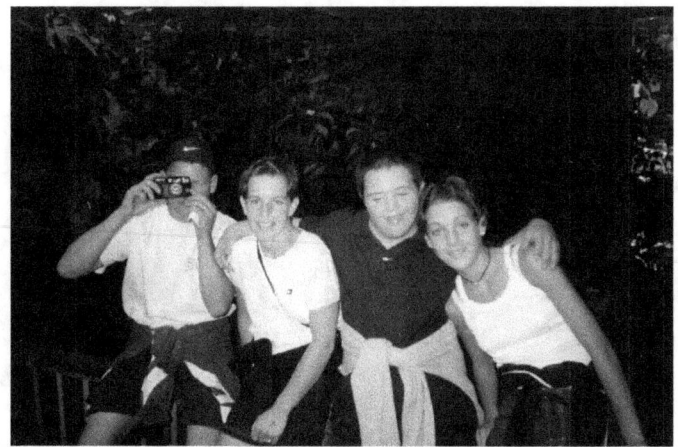

Chris, Shawna, Josh & Paula (Vacation in Banff)

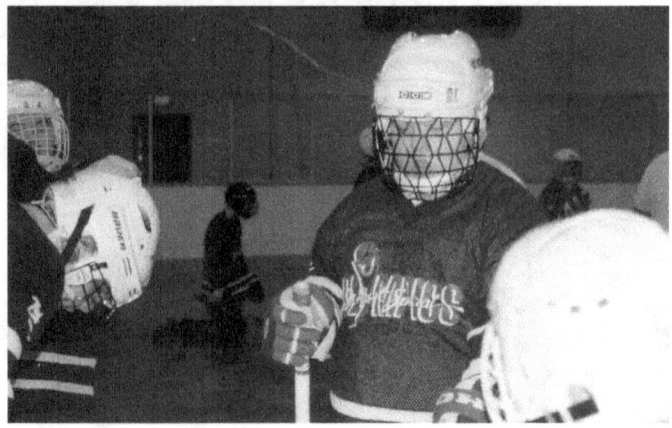

Josh Playing Floor Hockey – Special Olympics

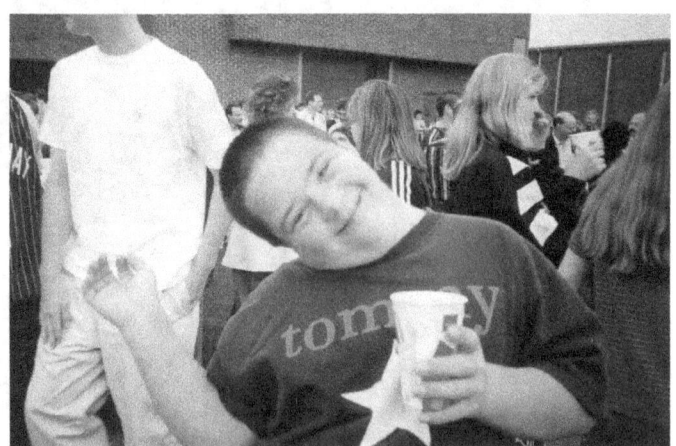

Josh The Clown – High School Years

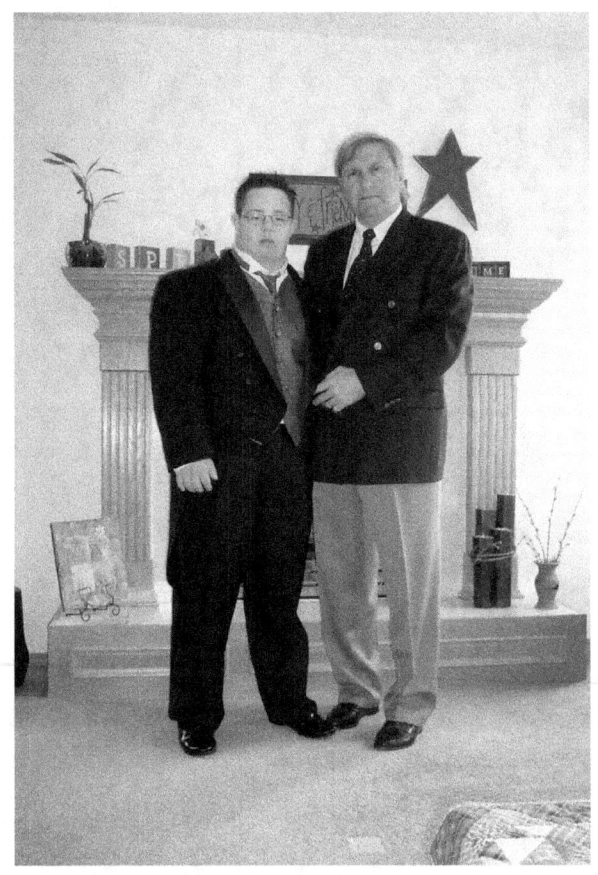

Josh & Joe (Grade 12 Graduation)

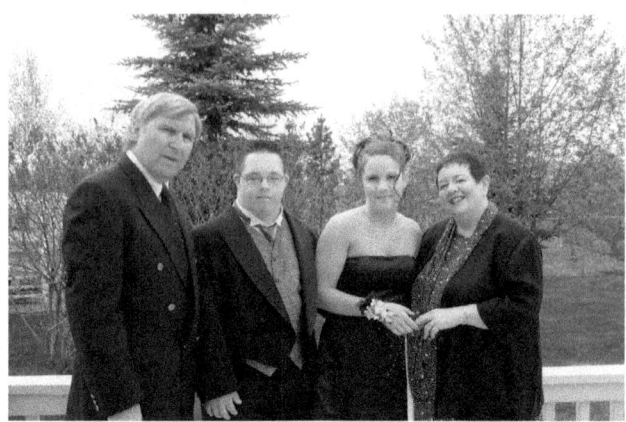

Joe, Josh, Megan, Karen (Grade 12 Graduation)

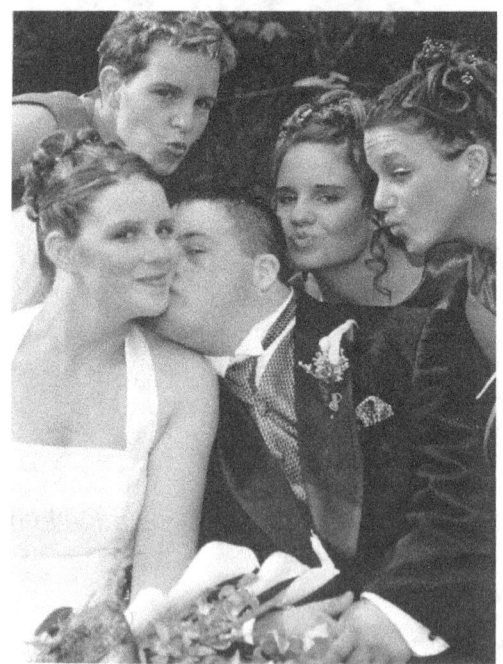

Josh at Jodie's Wedding (Jodie, Shawna, Josh, Megan & Paula)

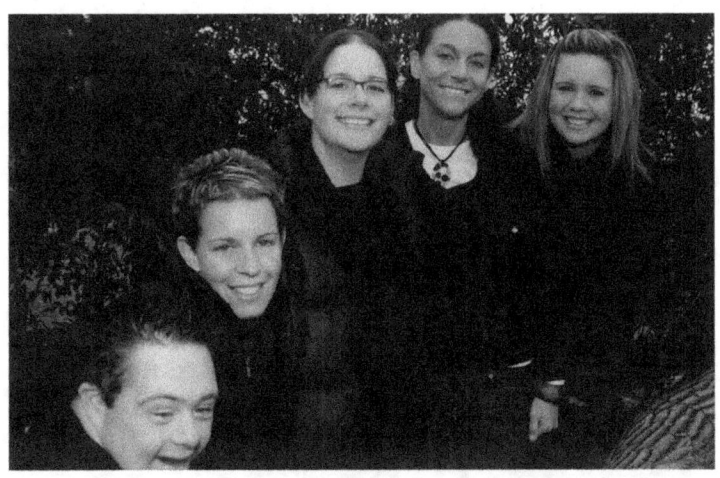

Josh, Shawna, Jodie, Paula, Megan

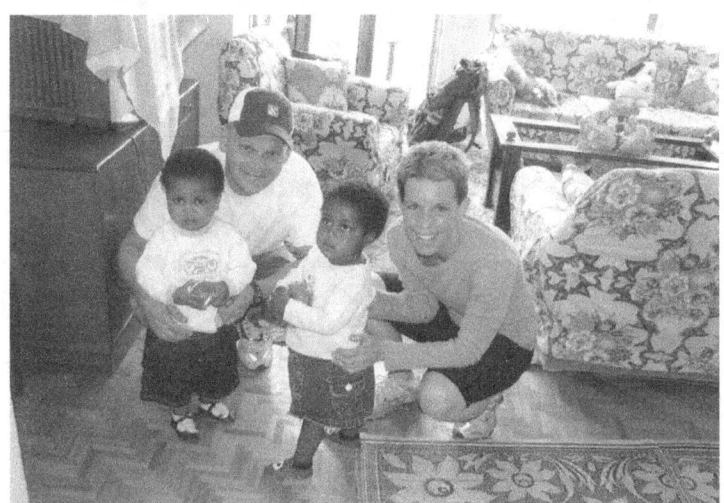

Chris & Shawna with newly adopted twins McKeely and Mea.

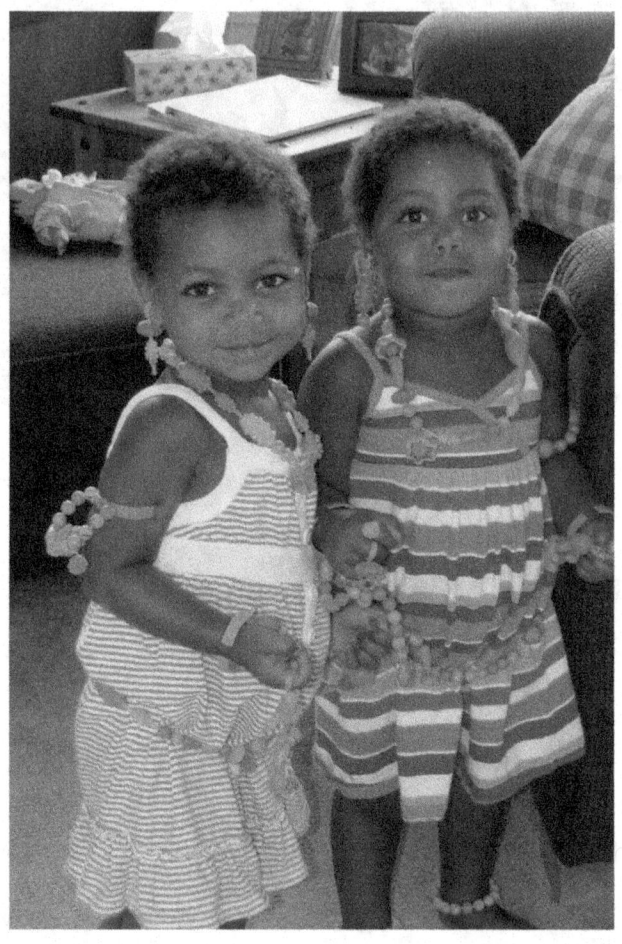

McKeely & Mea (Adopted Twins 1 year later)

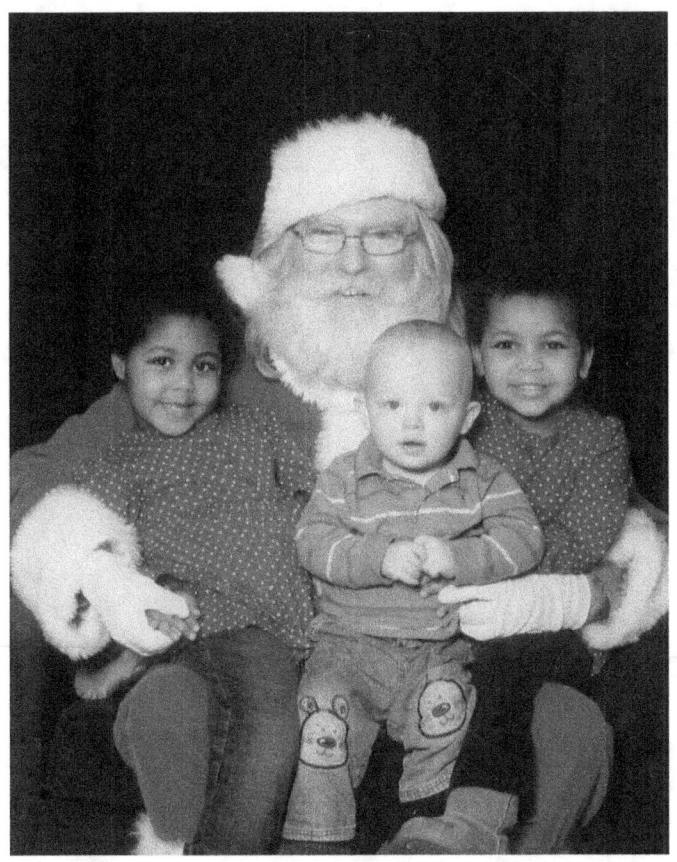

Mea, Luke and McKeely with Santa Claus

Can't Hold Me Down   Joe Petrone

ACKNOWLEDGEMENTS

I would like to thank my wife Karen for her heroic and tireless effort in Josh's upbringing and her total support for him. She is truly our family rock.

Thanks to my four wonderful daughters Shawna, Jodie, Paula and Megan as well as our son-in laws: Chris, Gage and Kent, for their unwavering support for Josh.

I would like to thank all his teachers, teacher aids especially Teresa Belland. St.Albert Special Olympic co-coordinator and mentor Wendy Stiver. A special thanks to Ian Klien, for his tireless volunteering of coaching expertise in floor hockey and soccer. Thanks also to the staff of the Alberta Special Olympics office and Carmen the director.

I would like to thank Alisa Makowksi for her technical knowledge and expertise in the development and setting of this book.

A special thanks to Carmelo & Stella Rago (Owners of Sorrentino's Restaurant Chain) for all their support of Special Olympics.

Special thanks to all our relatives, friends and neighbours who have helped to shape and work with Josh.

A special thanks to Julie Salembier for her support and editing expertise.

To John Ratcliffe for helping Josh to become a better floor hockey player, but most of all a better person.

ABOUT THE AUTHOR

Joe Petrone was born in Montagano, Campobasso, Italy, November 11th, 1945. He enrolled at St. Joseph's high school in Edmonton and played all major senior sports in all his high school years, which included soccer, basketball, volleyball and football (quarterback & place kicker). After graduation, he was the starting quarterback and kicker for the Edmonton Wildcats of the Alberta Junior Football league, and guided the team to the western finals for the first time in 1966.

Upon graduation, his talents amazed scouts in the US, not only for soccer, but football as well. He chose to accept a football scholarship with the Idaho State University. While being the quarterback and place kicker on the University team. Petrone kicked the longest field goal in the history of the Idaho State and the National Collegiate Athletics Association (NCAA) at the time of 59 yards. This tied Jan Stenarud's record set in 1965 with Montana State University.

After two years in the US, he boarded a northbound plane and headed back to Canada to continue to play soccer and football in this beautiful country of ours. He transferred to the University of Calgary in 1969 and was the top passer and scorer. Then after transferring to the University of Alberta in 1971 a few things happened that year. Not only was he the top scorer in the intercollegiate football league, he was a first round draft pick of the Calgary Stampeders. Petrone opted to sign a contract with the Dallas Cowboys of the NFL instead.

But in due time, soccer became more of a passion than football. Petrone continued to play soccer and played for the Canadian National team in the 1967 Pan AM games in Winnipeg and other national games. He was on the roster of the National Team program until 1974. Petrone also played for the Ital Canadians. With the ball back at his feet, he continued to excel, scoring over

400 goals in his career which ranked him as the top scorer in history of the Alberta Major Soccer league.

Then came 1979 when the soccer scene exploded and Petrone became an assistant coach, not long before moving to the ranks of head coach and general manager of the Edmonton Drillers of the NASL in 1980 to 1982. Moving forward and continuing his sports management career he became the General Manager of the Edmonton Eagles of the first Canadian Soccer League. One year later as a General Manager, the Edmonton Eagles would win the CSL Championship in 1983. Continuing his career in soccer, Petrone became the Director of Soccer Operations for the Edmonton Brickmen from 1987 to 1990 as well as for the Edmonton Drillers of the NPSL from 1996 to 2000. During his reign at the helm neither team ever missed the play-offs, with the exception of two teams which folded prior to the end of the season.

Petrone is a graduate of the University of Alberta with a Bachelor of Education and holds a Master's of Science Degree from the University of Eastern Illinois. He is married (Karen) with five children, Shawna, Jodie, Paula, Josh, and Megan. Petrone was a teacher in the Edmonton Catholic School board and a director of the soccer academy at Holy Trinity High School before retiring. He presently consults with soccer related activities in Canada.